# The Keto Vegan

## 87 Low-Carb Plant-Based Recipes for a Ketogenic Diet

*The Carbless Cook 4*
*By Lydia Miller*
*Version 1.0*
*Published by **veganvegetarianketo***

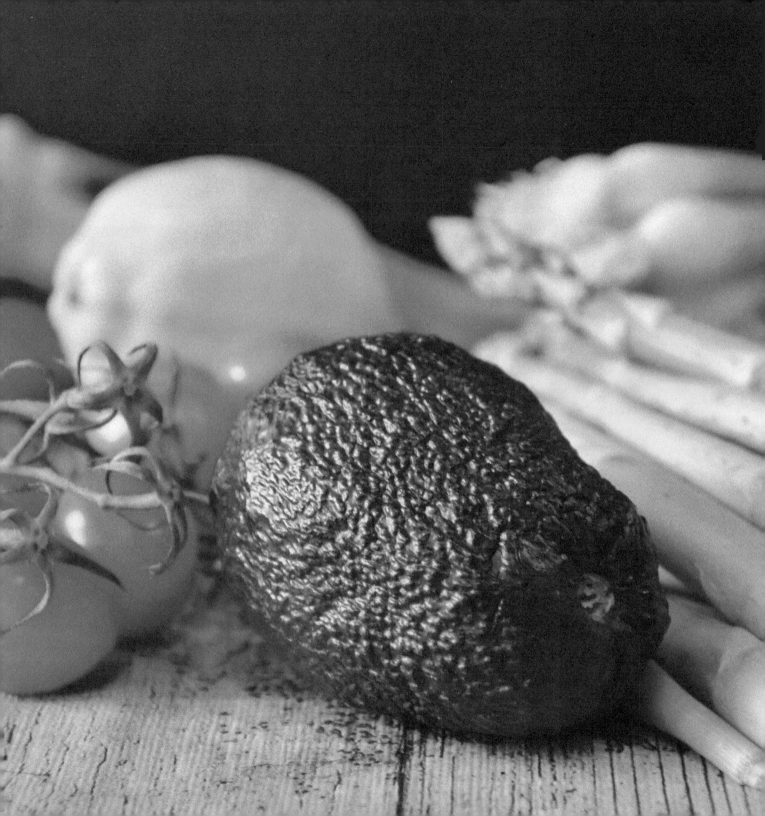

# Introduction

Ketogenic and plant-based diets have gained a lot of attention in recent years as a result of unprecedented chronic illness epidemics and a general shift toward a health-conscious way of life, as well as growing humanitarian and environmental concerns.

This book will serve as a guide to the low-carbohydrate high-fat (LCHF) plant-based diet, providing both background information and a range of recipes, which will aid the successful adoption of the diet.

The ketogenic vegan diet is exactly what is sounds like. It combines the ketogenic diet with the plant-based-, or for lack of better words, vegan diet. Vegans do not consume meat, fish, and other animal products. Many people choose to adopt this lifestyle for religious, moral, and/or health reasons.

There has been a lot of controversy surrounding the adoption of plant-based diets, and many people still believe that such diets are detrimental to one's health. Over the past 30 years, however, evidence has increasingly suggested that (mostly) plant-based diets are healthier than traditional western diets in which meat consumption is high, which results in high intake of saturated fat, cholesterol, calories, carcinogenic preservatives, salt, sugar, and chemical byproducts from the cooking process[1].

Guidelines have been established for those who wish to be able to successfully adopt plant-based diets in a healthy and responsible way. These include ensuring adequate intake of plant foods high in iron and protein, as well as supplementation[2] of some micronutrients such as vitamin B12.

The ketogenic diet, on the other hand, is based on the reduction of blood glucose through the restrictive consumption of carbohydrates, the energy source from which glucose is derived. Glucose typically serves as the body's main source of fuel so doing this results in the production of alternative energy sources by the liver's ketone bodies – a source of energy produced from the breakdown of stored fats. Studies have shown that the short-term effects of the ketogenic diet are weight loss, reductions of low-density lipoproteins (LDL), and blood triglycerides, which all lower the risk of cardiovascular diseases.

The ketogenic vegan diet is fat-based and allows for the consumption of plant fats, such as the fats found in vegetable oils, nuts, seeds and avocados.

The possibility of being able to improve your health while contributing to the betterment of the world, not to mention continuing to enjoy delicious food may seem too good to be true. With the help of this book, you will see how simple it is to accomplish this. Innocent animal lives and your health do not have to be sacrificed for good-tasting food. As you read through these chapters, you will find yourself letting go of outdated and questionable beliefs and embracing a new low-carb, guilt-free lifestyle!

# Table of Contents

3

# Snacks & Desserts

# Disclaimer

The recipes provided in this report are for informational purposes only and are not intended to provide dietary advice. A medical practitioner should be consulted before making any changes in your diet. Additionally, recipe cooking times may require adjustment depending on age and quality of appliances. Readers are strongly urged to take all precautions to ensure ingredients are fully cooked in order to avoid the dangers of foodborne viruses. The recipes and suggestions provided in this book are solely the opinion of the author. The author and publisher do not take any responsibility for any consequences that may result due to following the instructions provided in this book.

**Congratulations with your responsible and health-conscious decision to read my book.**

*I'm very excited for you!*

I offer my readers an *exclusive* opportunity to become part of my keto circle. Dozens of people are already inside and enjoying *extra* (vegan & vegetarian) keto-genic recipes and support on their journey to fat-fueled cooking, more energy and weight loss.

Join a growing number of 'plant-ketoers' and become part of my circle!

**https://forms.aweber.com/form/96/2128265096.htm**

You'll get *'The Keto Vegetarian: 8 Reader-Exclusive Low-Carb, Plant-Based, Egg & Dairy Recipes'* as a welcome gift!

Subscribe to my newsletter and join dozens of people with similar aims and ethics.

**https://forms.aweber.com/form/96/2128265096.htm**

*(I absolutely hate spam and will never email you more than twice a week.)*

As a member of my keto circle, you will receive some of my latest recipes, exclusive opportunities to get new releases free of charge, and more...!

As a member of my keto circle, you can also always reach out for personal questions!

Check out my Facebook page:

**www.facebook.com/veganvegetarianketo**

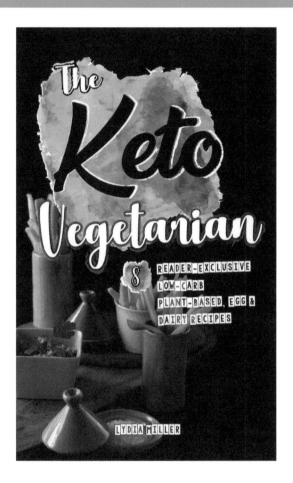

And our Facebook group**:**

**www.facebook.com/groups/veganvegetarianketo**

Where you get inspired, share results with other 'plant-ketoers' and stay motivated on your keto journey!

See you inside!

*Lydia*

# What is the Ketogenic Diet?

The typical proportional intake of macronutrients is around 45-65% carbohydrates, 20-35% fats, and 15-20% proteins. Carbohydrates are broken down more easily, which is why they serve as the body's primary source of fuel for immediate energy supply. Fat, on the other hand, is broken down less efficiently, so it is typically stored as an alternative fuel source for when glucose is not readily available. Proteins are used primarily for structural functions such as tissue repair and enzyme production and are only used as a source of fuel in a state of starvation.

In order to understand ketosis, it is important to understand the role of glucose beyond its function as an immediate source of energy derived from the digestion of carbohydrates. The body also converts excess glucose to glycogen, a long-term energy storage found in the liver and the muscles. Under caloric restriction, glycogen is converted back into glucose to keep glucose levels in the blood within the normal range. In muscle tissue, it is broken down on-site to provide energy for muscle activity.

If glycogen stores are depleted, the body will rely on protein and fat from the diet for energy. Most cell types can use fatty acids as a fuel source. Fat stores will also be broken down, leading to weight loss.

In order to induce the breakdown of fat, which goes hand in hand with ketosis, fewer carbs and more fat need to be consumed. The remaining carbohydrates should be complex, as these require more energy to be broken down and produce a more gradual release of glucose into the blood. Complex carbs are found in ingredients such as veggies, whole grains, beans, and lentils. On a strict ketogenic regime, protein is also restricted because it triggers the release of a growth factor that stimulates the uptake of glucose from the blood.[3]

As fatty acids are mobilized from adipose tissue (fat stores), the ketogenic pathway is activated in the liver, converting acetyl-CoA into ketone bodies, which are then used as fuel. Ketone bodies represent three water-soluble molecules: beta-hydroxybutyrate, acetoacetate, and acetone.

Ketogenic diets are effective in the short-term for weight loss and treatment of cardiovascular risk factors. Long-term, a more moderate diet such as a low-carb diet can be adopted in order to make it sustainable and avoid muscle loss.[4] It is crucial that the ketogenic diet is carried out correctly. Failure to do so can result in illness or other serious health problems. Long-term ketogenic diets prescribed by a dietician or doctor for medical reasons should be followed strictly according to his/her guidelines.

## Why eating more fat may lead to more fat being burned

There is ample evidence to suggest that fat loss occurs in people who adopt a ketogenic diet, however, there has been much debate as to the exact mechanisms behind these effects. One theory is that consumption of carbohydrates results in a rise of insulin in the bloodstream. Insulin is the hormone responsible for the uptake of glucose and fatty acids into tissue cells, including adipose cells that store fat. Insulin also suppresses the breakdown of fat (lipolysis). Therefore, when blood insulin levels are low, there is an overall increase in the buildup of fat stores.

This theory has been challenged by findings that insulin is not solely responsible for fat uptake. Acylation stimulating protein (ASP) is released in response to fat intake in the diet and potently increases fatty acid uptake into adipose cells.[5] There is also some debate as to whether insulin's effects are direct or whether uptake results from increased insulin release in response to ASP fat.[6] This could possibly explain why not everyone who undergoes a ketogenic diet loses weight.

Another theory is based on the fact that, following a rapid increase in insulin levels, there is a drop, which induces a hunger response. When these insulin spikes and drops are not occurring, appetite is more tightly regulated. Additionally, people on a ketogenic diet may experience higher levels of satiety from the protein and fat intake and the appetite suppressant action of ketone bodies themselves. Ultimately, this leads to lower calorie intake and eventual fat loss.

The hypothesis that weight loss occurs because protein and fat digestion are more "expensive," or use more energy, than the digestion of carbohydrates is also a popular theory. In the initial phases of the ketogenic diet, 16% of the glucose the body needs are produced by the body itself, through "gluconeogenesis," an energy-demanding process that converts glycerol and glycogenic amino acids from fat and protein into glucose. The energy required for this process comes from the breakdown of fat stores in the absence of glucose.[7]

## What is Veganism?

A vegan can be defined as "a person who does not eat meat or fish, and also avoids other animal products, especially for moral, religious, or health reasons." Being vegan is more than a dietary choice; it is often a lifestyle choice, which is usually made after a lot of thought and with strong motives.

Becoming a vegan, or following a plant-based diet, is a personal choice. One reason an individual may choose the vegan lifestyle is morality. Many believe it is unethical to produce meat, fish or other animal products because animals suffer in the process. Increasingly, people are choosing to follow plant-based diets out of concern for the environment, since raising livestock contributes to the release of greenhouse gases. It also requires vast amounts of farmland and energy and can harm quality of life in many farmland communities around the world. Some religions such as Jainism, Hinduism, and Buddhism either require or advocate vegetarianism or veganism as a moral obligation.

It is important to carefully monitor nutrient consumption on a vegan diet because some nutrients that are readily available in animal products are found in lower quantities in plants. One of the biggest concerns is adequate intake of protein. In the body, protein is broken down into its constituents, amino acids. Amino acids serve many vital functions; they are the structural components of many tissues and enzymes, which take part in biochemical processes critical to life.

# Macronutrients

Macronutrients are nutrients that our bodies require in large amounts to provide energy. The three macronutrients are proteins, carbohydrates, and fats. Each macronutrient provides a different amount of energy per gram.

- *1 g protein = 4 calories*
- *1 g carb = 4 calories*
- *1 g fat = 9 calories*

## Protein

The human body's structural components, including hair, nails, muscles, and organs, are all made up of protein. Protein from the diet is broken down into amino acids, which are then re-assimilated into protein structures. These structures are regularly undergoing repair. One example of such a protein structure is muscle, which is broken down during a workout, and repaired during the recovery period.

In addition to these structures, enzymes – proteins responsible for making chemical reactions in the body efficient – and antibodies – proteins responsible for the prevention of infection and disease – are also dependent on protein derived from the diet.

It is clear that protein is vital for the body to function normally. If not enough protein is present in the diet, the body enters a "starvation" mode and begins breaking down muscle fiber. It is therefore vital to consume sufficient protein.

It is important to note that while on a ketogenic diet, protein can act as an alternative source of glucose.

Because it is the most efficient energy source in the absence of carbohydrates, the body will seek to convert any extra protein available into glucose through a process called gluconeogenesis. Although this scenario is unlikely, since protein is less abundant in most plant sources in comparison to meat and fish, consuming too much protein can prevent ketosis even while following the ketogenic diet.[8]

## Amino Acids

Amino acids are the building blocks of life. Individual amino acids serve essential functions. For example, tryptophan plays a role in the synthesis of serotonin, which regulates your mood, while arginine is used in the synthesis of nitric oxide to facilitate cardiovascular health.

Amino acids establish peptide bonds between them to form peptides and then polypeptides, which combine to make the protein structures that are a part of all the crucial chemical reactions that take place in your body, contributing to reproduction, metabolism, immunity, cell signaling, cell growth and differentiation, gene expression, anti-oxidative defense, and protein synthesis.[9]

Twenty different kinds of amino acids are used to create proteins. Nine of the amino acids are known as "essential amino acids". These amino acids (methionine, leucine, isoleucine, histidine, lysine, phenylalanine, tryptophan, valine, and threonine) cannot be synthesized in the body and must be obtained from nutrition. The other amino acids (alanine, arginine, asparagine, aspartate/aspartic acid, cysteine, glutamine, glutamate/glutamic acid, glycine, proline, serine, and tyrosine) are classified as non-essential.[10]

As non-essential amino acids are produced by the body from essential amino acids, it is important to ensure the required intake for all essential amino acids. If you don't consume the required levels of protein from which the essential amino acids are derived, a condition called hyperproteinemia (tissue degradation) can occur. As protein is more concentrated in meat and fish, the most common protein sources in typical western diets, being vegan requires extra vigilance to ensure all amino acids are acquired through a combination of diverse protein sources.[11] Part of your body's mass is made up of protein, and amino acids carry out key bodily functions. An individual weighing 70kg generally has a protein make-up of around 12kg. These two numbers are used to calculate individual nutritional requirements to maintain body weight and monitor your plasma protein levels.[12]

Plant proteins are less bioavailable to humans than animal proteins, but still comprise a great source of protein. Soya is one protein source that provides all essential amino acids.[13] Exact recommended protein intake varies from country to country, however the estimated protein needs, according to the *American Journal of Clinical Nutrition*, are roughly 0.6g per kilogram of body weight.[14]

## The importance of Lysine

Lysine is one of the nine essential amino acids previously mentioned. It plays a crucial role as a building block of proteins. Lysine is needed for growth, as well as energy conversion and cholesterol level maintenance. This amino acid is converted in the human body to acetyl-CoA, which is a key factor in carbohydrate metabolism and energy production. It is also a precursor of carnitine, another amino acid responsible for the transportation of fatty acids that are used for energy production. Carnitine also has the ability to induce strong inflammatory and immune responses and plays a role in healing wounds and in inducing extensive angiogenic responses.[15] Symptoms of a carnitine deficiency include:

- Fatigue
- Nausea
- Dizziness
- Anorexia
- Slow growth
- Anemia

## How much Lysine do you need and how can you get it?

According to a joint report from the *World Health Organization*, the *Food and Agriculture Organization*, and *United Nations University*[16], *30mg lysine per 1 kg of body weight should be consumed on a daily basis. This means approximately 2.1g for an individual weighing 70 kg. Vegans can get lysine from foods such as nuts and soy products like tofu. Lysine deficiency is rare, and it is important to note that a sharp rise in lysine amino acids in the body can lead to an increase in cholesterol and upset the stomach.*

## Lysine-rich vegan protein sources

Lysine is found in large amounts in meat and poultry, but there are also a wide variety of vegan options. Foods that contain high amounts of lysine include tempeh, tofu, soymilk, black beans and pistachios.

| | | |
|---|---|---|
| **Tempeh** | 30g protein/cup | 754mg lysine |
| **Black beans** | 14g protein/cup | 1046mg lysine |
| **Soymilk** | 9g protein/cup | 439mg lysine |
| **Pistachios** | 12g protein/cup | 734mg lysine |
| **Seitan** | 6.7g protein/oz | 219mg lysine |

## Carbohydrates

Carbohydrate molecules comprised of hydrogen, carbon, and oxygen are, as previously discussed, the body's preferred source of energy-efficient glucose.

Carbohydrates commonly found in the diet are sugar, fiber, and starch. Foods rich in carbohydrates are cheap to purchase and activate the body's reward system upon ingestion, which is why they are so popular. Many of the most commonly available carbohydrates lack micronutrients and serve simply as an energy source.

That said, not all carbohydrates are created equal. There are two types of carbohydrates: simple and complex. Simple carbohydrates, also known as simple sugars, are easily broken down during digestion because they are only made up of one or two units of sugar linked by glycosidic bonds. These include monosaccharides (glucose, fructose, and galactose) and disaccharides (sucrose, and maltose).[17]

Simple carbohydrates fall into the category of high-glycemic index foods that cause a rapid rise in blood sugar levels and subsequent insulin release. Examples of high-glycemic index foods are sodas, juices, and foods that include highly processed (refined) carbohydrates such as white bread, pasta, rice, breakfast cereals, crackers, pretzels, sweets, and desserts.[18]

Complex carbohydrates are typically low- or medium-glycemic index foods and facilitate a much more gradual release of sugar into the bloodstream after the consumption of a meal. This is because it takes longer to digest the oligosaccharide and polysaccharide chains that make up complex carbs. Examples of complex carbohydrate foods are whole wheat bread, oats, sweet potatoes/yams, corn, beans, peas and legumes, most fruits, as well as non-starchy vegetables like carrots.

Complex carbs do not cause rapid insulin spikes and keep you satiated longer since they sit in the gut for longer periods of time during the digestion process. This leads to less frequent food intake, which ultimately results in less energy being stored as fat.

Consume more complex carbs than simple carbs. If you are following a gluten-free regimen, sources such as lentils, beans, and green peas are best.

## Fats

Although fat has gotten a bad rep in the media over the past few decades, fat is actually a crucial component of our diet. Fat plays a vital role in the functioning of cells. We also need fat to absorb the fat-soluble vitamins A, D, E, and K. The macronutrient also serves as an insulator and offers protective functions to internal organs.

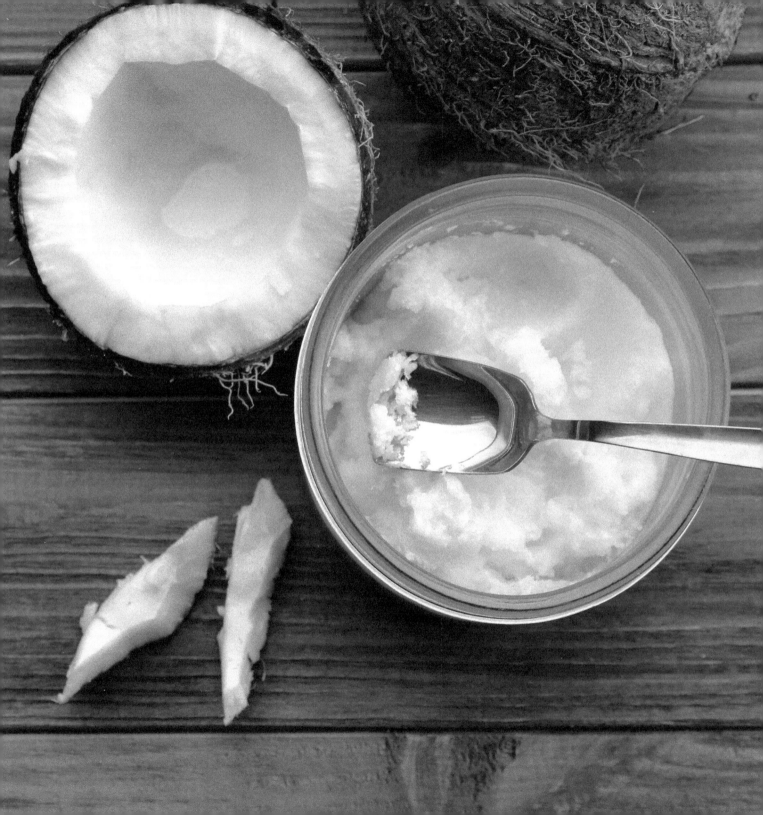

Dietary fat is typically divided into two broader categories: saturated and unsaturated fats, with the latter being the healthier option due to their structures. They contain at least one double bond between their carbon molecules (monounsaturated) but often contain more (polyunsaturated). This introduces kinks in their carbon and hydrogen structures and gives them certain properties, like being liquid at room temperature, while saturated fats are solid.

Consuming too much saturated fat can cause high cholesterol levels, which lead to health complications such as cardiovascular disease. Vegan sources of saturated fat are typically nuts, seeds and canola oil. Unsaturated fats are found in avocados, nuts, seeds, and vegetable oils.

Olive oil, which offers several health benefits and can withstand high temperatures when heated, is a great, affordable source of fat.[19] In comparison with butter and coconut oil, olive oil contains higher levels of monounsaturated fats than saturated fats and is the better option for those on a vegan diet.[20]

Other vegetable oils such as palm oil offer a more neutral contribution to the blood lipid profile. Despite containing high amounts of saturated fats, some of these oils, such as palmitic acid, have similar effects on the lipid profile as monounsaturated fats and contain cholesterol-lowering compounds.[21]

A third category of fat that should be avoided at all costs is trans-fat. This is an unsaturated type of fat that is chemically hydrogenated into saturated fats to give them certain properties such as spreadability and an extended shelf life. The consumption of trans-fat increases the amount of harmful LDL cholesterol in the blood. It also reduces the beneficial HDL-levels. Avoid trans-fat even in the smallest amounts, as only 2% of daily calories derived from these fats can increase the risk to heart diseases by 23%.

## Coconut Oil

As mentioned above, plant-based fats are key components for meeting fat needs in a vegan diet. One of these sources is coconut oil, which has been promoted for consumption and other uses in recent years. While coconut oil offers a very distinct and full flavor, the nutritional properties have been exaggerated.

The available evidence that coconut oil lowers cardiovascular risk factors is weak, and there has been no clear indication that it improves lipid profiles. Reviews of the available literature suggest that unsaturated fats are a much better option when attempting to lower CVD risk.[22] Substitutes such as olive oil, hemp seed oil, and flax seed oil are better options to improve your lipid profile.

# Healthy Oils and Fats

Perhaps the most significance reason to get the right balance of unsaturated and saturated fat in your diet is to optimize your blood lipid profile. A poor profile is a key risk factor in the development of metabolic syndrome, which is a cluster of biochemical and physiological abnormalities associated with the development of cardiovascular disease and type 2 diabetes. The consumption of monounsaturated and polyunsaturated fats contribute to the elevation of high-density lipoproteins (HDL) in the blood. This is often referred to as "good" cholesterol.

There has been a lot of controversy around the optimal intake levels of different fats. More recent studies have suggested that merely reducing the intake of "bad" cholesterol, or low-density lipoproteins, does not reduce an individual's coronary risk factor if HDL levels remain low. Insufficient omega-3 intake in particular carries a high cardiovascular disease burden.[23]

Besides keeping blood lipid profiles in balance, omega-3 fatty acids play a role in aiding brain function and in preventing asthma, certain cancers, and arthritis. While omega-3 fatty acids are most commonly found in fatty fish such as salmon and sardines, it is perfectly doable to satisfy your body's needs with vegan foods like chia, flax or hemp seeds, flaxseed oils, brussels sprouts, and various nuts.

Getting the right ratio of omega-6s to omega-3s is important. Unlike omega-9s, these two fats cannot be produced by the body and must be derived from the diet in a ratio. The ideal ratio of 1:1 prevents inflammation, which is caused by higher intake of pro-inflammatory omega-6s.

According to various studies, 95 % of Americans [24] have dangerously unbalanced omega-6 to omega-3 ratios, at around 15:1. Even an imbalance as small as 10:1 shows adverse health effects. With more careful monitoring of your diet, you will be able to achieve a more appropriate intake ratio through consumption of whole foods. Omega-6s can be found in seeds, nuts, green veggies, and oils, such as olive oil.

To recap, consciously consuming foods such as flaxseed oil, hemp seeds, chia seeds, walnuts, and algal oil that are higher in omega-3s, which are less abundant in typical western diets, will help you to remain in balance.[25]

Omega-9 fatty acids are a non-essential fatty acid, since the body can produce these by itself. Their production is dependent on sufficient levels of omega-6s and omega-3s, though they can also be obtained from avocados, nuts, chia seeds, and olive oil.

Since fats are energy-dense, overconsumption of any fat will result in energy imbalance and weight gain. The amount of energy taken in should be equal to or less than the energy expended. Everything in moderation!

## Keto-Flu and Mineral Deficiencies

In the initial phases of the keto diet journey, there is the possibility of experiencing "keto-flu" owed to the effects of the drop in carbohydrate intake. It is crucial at this stage to carefully monitor electrolyte intake. A lack of magnesium and potassium can cause lethargy and, in extreme cases, lead to heart dysfunction.

## Potassium

The consumption of 3500 to 4700mg potassium per day potassium is recommended. A potassium deficiency can lead to hypokalemia, cardiac arrhythmia, muscle cramps, weakness, and anorexia. An avocado, which is low-carb, provides roughly 1000 mg of potassium. Spinach, zucchini and cauliflower are also great keto-vegan potassium sources.

Depending on food sources, supplementing potassium is recommended on a ketogenic vegan diet. It should also be noted that too much potassium could be toxic, potentially causing hyperkalemia.

## Magnesium

Adult males should be consuming around 320-420mg magnesium per day. For adult females, the recommended amount per day is 300-400mg. Magnesium contributes to protein synthesis, the metabolism of glucose, muscle contraction, bone structure, and bone strength. The consumption of less than 300mg per day for an extended period can cause magnesium deficiency, resulting in muscle weakness and cramps, as well as cardiac arrhythmia.

Good natural sources of this mineral are nuts, cacao, soy products, and dark, leafy greens. Supplementing is good idea if you're struggling to get sufficient magnesium from your diet, but be aware that a maximum of 350 mg/day of magnesium in supplement form is tolerable.

The consumption of magnesium in large amounts is possibly unsafe. Symptoms of toxicity are nausea, vomiting and diarrhea.

## Sodium

The recommended intake of sodium is roughly 1500mg per day for the body to regulate its water and acid-base balance and to guarantee nerve functioning and muscle contraction. Symptoms of a deficiency include hyponatremia, nausea, anorexia, seizures, and in the worst cases, a coma.

Some keto-vegan sodium sources include pickles, soy sauce, and salt, like Maldon, Himalayan, or table salt. It is just as important to get enough sodium as to avoid too much sodium, which can put your body at risk for kidney stones and some types of cancer.

## Calcium

It is commonly known that calcium is important for the structure and strength of bones and teeth. Calcium also contributes to a healthy acid-base balance and takes part in nerve function, muscle contraction, blood clotting, and enzyme activation. Aim to consume roughly 1000mg per day. Great low-carb calcium sources include soy products, leafy vegetables, and almonds.

## Zinc

Zinc plays an important role in protein synthesis, energy metabolism, immune functions, sensory functions, and the production of sex hormones. Women should aim to take in roughly 8mg per day, while males should aim for 11mg. Sources include seeds, nuts, legumes and nutritional yeast.

## Iron

Iron is one of the most important dietary minerals because it plays a crucial role in oxygen delivery and is an essential component of the aerobic metabolism. Unfortunately, it is one of the more common deficiencies, particularly in women, vegetarians, and vegans.

An iron deficiency is more common in vegans because iron from plant sources is less easily absorbed into the blood stream. It is important to ensure adequate vitamin C intake because this vitamin facilitates the absorption of iron in the gut. Common low-carb sources of vitamin C include bell peppers, broccoli, strawberries, lemons, and dark, leafy greens.

The average iron needs for males is roughly 8mg per day while the requirement for females is closer to 18mg per day, for proper functioning of the menstrual cycle. Good vegan sources include legumes, nuts, seeds, dark, leafy greens and small portions of dried fruit. Due to the poor absorption rates of iron from plant-based sources, consider iron supplements.

Note that polyphenols, phytates, and calcium can decrease the amount of iron absorbed. These elements are found in drinks life coffee and tea, and in grains and legumes. If you have an iron deficiency, it is best to avoid iron-containing ingredients that are also high in elements that compete with iron for absorption.

## Iodine

Iodine is important for thyroid function. A deficiency is rarely a problem due to salt being fortified with Iodine. Most adults don't have trouble meeting the 150mg daily requirement, though in rare instances, severe deficiency can cause goiter.

## Phosphorus

Phosphorus requirements are roughly 700mg per day. This micronutrient promotes bone structure and strength, acid-base balance, and B-vitamin function. It is a component of the primary carrier of ATP, which stores and transports energy in cells. Sources include high-protein foods such as tofu, legumes, and nuts. A deficiency is unlikely since small amounts are also found in vegetables and fruits.

## Vitamin B12

The B12 vitamin is needed for important bodily functions such as protein metabolism and synthesis, fat and carbohydrate metabolism, neurotransmitter formation, and glycolysis. Vitamin B12 is difficult to obtain on a vegan diet. Like complete amino acid profiles, it is more commonly found in meat and fish. Eggs, milk and cheese also contain B12, but in low quantities and it tends to be poorly absorbed.

Supplementation of B12 is a smart choice for vegans. Also, foods such almond milk are often fortified with vitamin B12. Consuming these fortified products can help to ensure adequate intake, which is roughly 2.4-2.5mg per day.

A deficiency of vitamin B12 could lead to pernicious anemia, particularly in elderly people who have more trouble absorbing the vitamin. Being knowledgeable about vitamin B12 requirements and its functions will guard your health while following a ketogenic-vegan diet.

# The Ketogenic Vegan Diet in Numbers

A ketogenic vegan diet, simply put, is fat-rich and plant-based. The consumption of carbohydrates on a ketogenic diet are minimized. A combination of both diets is slightly more challenging than the ordinary ketogenic diet, in which meat and fish can also be consumed for low-carb protein and fat.

To maintain a state of ketosis, the number of net carbs you can consume each day is limited to a recommended 30g. In order to achieve this, a strict meal plan is necessary. It is possible to consume up to 50g of carbohydrates and still lose weight, but this depends on calorie intake and goals of the individual. Since weight loss requires a calorie deficit, those aiming to lose bodyfat need to monitor calorie intake as well.

The following is a breakdown of the percentages of macronutrients needed to formulate your diet more accurately:
- *5-10% of calories should come from carbs.*
- *15-30% of calories should come from protein.*
- *60-75% of calories should come from fatty foods.*

## Fiber & Net Carbs

It is important to take a close look at the effects of fiber on blood glucose levels. There are two types of fiber: soluble fiber and insoluble fiber. The first can lower cholesterol levels and improve blood glucose[26], and the second keeps the digestive tract working well. You should aim to consume about 14 grams of fiber for every 1,000 calories to provide your body with these benefits. Foods like Chia seeds, berries, avocado, almonds, and various vegetables make it easy to obtain enough fiber from a keto-vegan diet.

Most people think that fiber does not affect blood sugar levels and that it doesn't contain calories. That's why many people only count the "net carbs" in a ketogenic dish: total carbs minus the fiber content. However, the US Food and Drug Administration (FDA) estimates that each gram of soluble fiber fermented by bacteria provides about 2 calories[27]. Insoluble fibers are not digested at all, so the FDA estimates that they do not contribute any calories.

# Low-Carb Vegan Foods

## Carbs in nuts & seeds

If you make the decision to follow a ketogenic-vegan diet, it is useful to know the nutritional values of different nuts and seeds, as they tend to have fewer carbohydrates than other plant-based foods. They make a nice, portable snack, but be selective in choosing which to include in your diet, as a few are high in carbs (chestnuts, pistachios, and cashews).

The serving size has been set to 1 ounce to make it easy to calculate a larger serving.

| Food | Serving | Fats(g) | Carbs(g) | Fiber(g) | Protein(g) | Net Carbs(g) |
|------|---------|---------|----------|----------|------------|--------------|
| Chia seed | 1 oz | 9 | 12 | 11 | 4 | 1 |
| Pecan | 1 oz | 20 | 4 | 3 | 3 | 1 |
| Flax Seed | 1 oz | 12 | 8 | 7 | 5 | 1 |
| Brazil Nut | 1 oz | 19 | 4 | 2 | 4 | 2 |
| Hazelnut | 1 oz | 17 | 5 | 3 | 4 | 2 |
| Walnut | 1 oz | 18 | 4 | 2 | 4 | 2 |
| Coconut, Unsweetened | 1 oz | 18 | 7 | 5 | 2 | 2 |
| Macadamia Nut | 1 oz | 21 | 4 | 2 | 2 | 2 |
| Almond | 1 oz | 15 | 5 | 3 | 6 | 2 |
| Almond Flour | 1 oz | 14 | 6 | 3 | 6 | 3 |
| Pumpkin Seed | 1 oz | 6 | 4 | 1 | 10 | 3 |
| Sesame Seed | 1 oz | 14 | 7 | 3 | 5 | 4 |
| Sunflower Seed | 1 oz | 14 | 7 | 3 | 6 | 4 |

# Carbs in greens

Vegetables are the staple food of a healthy plant-based diet. Not all vegetables are low in carbohydrates, so it is important make sure to select the right ones. Avoid those high in sugar and starch, and take extra caution with some greens, which can add a surprising amount of carbs to your diet if you do not monitor your intake.

| Food | Serving | Metric | Fats(g) | Carbs(g) | Fiber(g) | Protein(g) | Net Carbs(g) |
|---|---|---|---|---|---|---|---|
| Endive | 2 oz. | 56g | 0 | 2 | 2 | 1 | 0 |
| Butter head Lettuce | 2 oz | 56g | 0 | 1 | 0.5 | 1 | 0.5 |
| Chicory | 2 oz | 56g | 0 | 2.5 | 2 | 1 | 0.5 |
| Beet Greens | 2 oz | 56g | 0 | 2.5 | 2 | 1 | 0.5 |
| Bok Choy | 2 oz | 56g | 0 | 1 | 0.5 | 1 | 0.5 |
| Alfalfa Sprouts | 2 oz | 56g | 0 | 2 | 1 | 2 | 1 |
| Spinach | 2 oz | 56g | 0 | 2 | 1 | 1.5 | 1 |
| Swiss Chard | 2 oz | 56g | 0 | 2 | 1 | 1 | 1 |
| Arugula | 2 oz | 56g | 0 | 2 | 1 | 1.5 | 1 |
| Celery | 2 oz | 56g | 0 | 2 | 1 | 0.5 | 1 |
| Chives | 2 oz | 56g | 0 | 2.5 | 1.5 | 2 | 1 |
| Collard Greens | 2 oz | 56g | 0 | 3 | 2 | 1.5 | 1 |
| Romaine lettuce | 2 oz | 56g | 0 | 2 | 1 | 1 | 1 |
| Asparagus | 2 oz | 56g | 0 | 2 | 1 | 1 | 1 |
| Eggplant | 2 oz | 56g | 0 | 3 | 2 | 0.5 | 1 |
| Radishes | 2 oz | 56g | 0 | 2 | 1 | 0.5 | 1 |
| Tomatoes | 2 oz | 56g | 0 | 2 | 1 | 0.5 | 1 |
| White mushrooms | 2 oz | 56g | 0 | 2 | 0.5 | 2 | 1.5 |
| Cauliflower | 2 oz | 56g | 0 | 3 | 1.5 | 1 | 1.5 |
| Cucumber | 2 oz | 56g | 0 | 2 | 0.5 | 0.5 | 1.5 |
| Dill pickles | 2 oz | 56g | 0 | 2 | 0.5 | 0.5 | 1.5 |

| Food | Serving | Metric | Fats(g) | Carbs(g) | Fiber(g) | Protein(g) | Net Carbs(g) |
|------|---------|--------|---------|----------|----------|------------|--------------|
| Bell green pepper | 2 oz | 56g | 0 | 2.5 | 1 | 0.5 | 1.5 |
| Cabbage | 2 oz | 56g | 0 | 3 | 1 | 1 | 2 |
| Fennel | 2 oz | 56g | 0 | 4 | 2 | 1 | 2 |
| Broccoli | 2 oz | 56g | 0 | 3.5 | 1.5 | 1.5 | 2 |
| Green Beans | 2 oz | 56g | 0 | 4 | 2 | 1 | 2 |
| Bamboo Shoots | 2 oz | 56g | 0 | 3 | 1 | 1.5 | 2 |

## Carbohydrates in fruits

The fruit of a plant is the reproductive organ that contains seeds. They are a popular food choice due their sweet taste. Okra, avocado, tomatoes, and green beans are in fact fruits, though many might think of them as vegetables. Avocados are an invaluable part of any keto diet as they are high in fat and low in carbohydrates.

| Food | Serving | Metric | Fats(g) | Carbs(g) | Fiber(g) | Protein(g) | Net Carbs(g) |
|------|---------|--------|---------|----------|----------|------------|--------------|
| Rhubarb | 2 oz | 56g | 0 | 2.5 | 1 | 1 | 1.5 |
| Lemon Juice | 1 oz | 28g | 0 | 2 | 0 | 0 | 2 |
| Lime Juice | 1 oz | 28g | 0 | 2 | 0 | 0 | 2 |
| Raspberries | 2 oz | 56g | 0 | 7 | 4 | 1 | 3 |
| Blackberries | 2 oz | 56g | 0 | 6 | 3 | 1 | 3 |
| Strawberries | 2 oz | 56g | 0 | 4 | 1 | 0 | 3 |

## Protein-rich vegan foods

| Food | Serving | Metric | Fats(g) | Carbs(g) | Fiber(g) | Protein(g) | Net Carbs(g) |
|------|---------|--------|---------|----------|----------|------------|--------------|
| Tofu | 3.5 oz | 100g | 5 | 2 | 1 | 16 | 1 |
| Pumpkin seed | 1 oz | 28g | 6 | 4 | 1 | 10 | 3 |
| Almond | 1 oz | 28g | 15 | 5 | 3 | 6 | 2 |
| Flax Seed | 1 oz | 28g | 12 | 8 | 7 | 5 | 1 |

| Food | Serving | Metric | Fats(g) | Carbs(g) | Fiber(g) | Protein(g) | Net Carbs(g) |
|------|---------|--------|---------|----------|----------|------------|--------------|
| Chia Seed | 1 oz | 28g | 9 | 12 | 11 | 4 | 1 |
| Brazil nut | 1 oz | 28g | 19 | 4 | 2 | 4 | 2 |
| Hazelnut | 1 oz | 28g | 17 | 5 | 3 | 4 | 2 |
| Walnut | 1 oz | 28g | 18 | 4 | 2 | 4 | 2 |
| Pecan | 1 oz | 28g | 20 | 4 | 3 | 3 | 1 |
| Unsweetened Coconut | 1 oz | 28g | 18 | 7 | 5 | 2 | 2 |
| Macadamia nut | 1 oz | 28g | 21 | 4 | 2 | 2 | 2 |

## Fat-rich vegan foods

As previously explained, monounsaturated and poly-unsaturated fats guarantee good cholesterol in the blood stream and should make up the majority of fats you consume. Remember that some saturated fat is needed, but in smaller amounts than unsaturated fat. Avoid trans-fat completely.

| Food | Serving | Metric | Fats(g) | Carbs(g) | Fiber(g) | Protein(g) | Net Carbs(g) |
|------|---------|--------|---------|----------|----------|------------|--------------|
| Avocado oil | 1 oz | 28g | 28 | 0 | 0 | 0 | 0 |
| Cocoa butter | 1 oz | 28g | 28 | 0 | 0 | 0 | 0 |
| Coconut oil | 1 oz | 28g | 28 | 0 | 0 | 0 | 0 |
| Flaxseed oil | 1 oz | 28g | 28 | 0 | 0 | 0 | 0 |
| Macadamia oil | 1 oz | 28g | 28 | 0 | 0 | 0 | 0 |
| MCT oil | 1 oz | 28g | 28 | 0 | 0 | 0 | 0 |
| Olive oil | 1 oz | 28g | 28 | 0 | 0 | 0 | 0 |
| Red palm oil | 1 oz | 28g | 28 | 0 | 0 | 0 | 0 |
| Coconut cream | 1 oz | 28g | 10 | 2 | 1 | 1 | 1 |
| Olives, green | 1 oz | 28g | 4 | 1 | 1 | 0 | 0 |
| Avocado | 1 oz | 28g | 4 | 2 | 2 | 1 | 0 |

# Losing Weight with a Ketogenic Vegan Diet

In order to lose weight, you must aim and maintain a calorie deficit. This means burning more energy than you consume. A typical female will consume around 1700 calories daily when dieting, and for men this figure will be roughly 2200, though the ideal target of course differs according to an individual's height, weight, and activity level.

To calculate how many daily calories you should be consuming, take the following steps:

1) Calculate your basal metabolic rate (BMR) using the following formula:

- For men: BMR = (9.99 x weight in kilograms) + (6.25 x height in centimeters) - 4.92 x age in years + 5. For women: BMR = (9.99 x weight in kilograms) + (6.25 x height in centimeters) - (4.92 x age in years) - 161.

2) Multiply your BMR by your activity factor:

- If you engage in no exercise your activity factor is 1.2.
- If you exercise one to three times a week, your activity factor is 1.375.
- If you exercise three to five times per week, your activity factor is 1.55.
- If you engage in heavy exercise six to seven times a week your activity factor is 1.72.
- If you are an athlete or train heavily for sport and/or have a physically demanding job, your activity factor is 1.9.

*The number you derive from this second calculation is the number of daily calories (kcal) you require to maintain your weight.*

3) Take the figure you obtained from the calculation in step 2 and subtract 500kcal. The number you get will be the number of calories you should be consuming per week in order to lose roughly 0.5kg of fat in a week.

Consuming less than this would be irresponsible. The effects of consuming too few calories can wreak havoc on your body. When you suddenly start consuming much less than your body is used to, it can kick into "starvation mode" and start breaking down muscle instead of fat in an effort to ensure the body's needs are met. This muscle loss will also show up as weight loss on the scale, but it goes without saying that this is not the goal you are attempting to achieve. Avoid retaining your excess fat and lose muscle.

Below are some guidelines to help ensure you are not consuming too many calories for the keto-vegan diet:

- Be sure to combat cravings by taking advantage of the satiating effects of protein.
- Avoid making the mistake of snacking on too many nuts, seeds, and other fat-rich nibbles when trying to lose weight. These foods are very calorie-dense.
- If you have not seen any clear weight loss results after 2-3 weeks, you should consider monitoring your calorie intake closely.
- Enjoy the many non-starchy vegetables such as cauliflower, spinach, kale, broccoli, zucchini, and bell peppers, as well as fruits like avocados or berries. These contain many micronutrients in addition to being low in carbs.
- Drink water throughout the day the hydrate the body and fill the stomach.

# How to test for ketosis

The body doesn't start burning fat as fuel the moment you lower your carb intake. That's why you want to start by aiming for nutritional ketosis. Once your body becomes fat-adapted, which happens after it has drained glycogen stores, it will start using fat as its main energy source.

As a rule, especially at first, no more than five percent of your calories should come from carbohydrates. This means no more than 20g of net carbs on a 1600 kcal diet or 25g of net carbs on a 2000 kcal diet.

To guarantee ketosis, these strict numbers are not always required. After the first days or week of careful carb restriction, ketosis kicks in, and there will be some room for flexibility. Obviously, this doesn't mean reintroducing as many carbs as you want. To make sure your body maintains a state of ketosis, use the following testing methods.

Checking for acetate, acetoacetate, and beta-hydroxybutyrate can be done by testing your blood, breath, and urine. The preferred method is to test your urine using keto strips. Eventually, you'll find your optimal level where you feel best and notice progress.

To be absolutely sure, test your blood. By measuring millimoles per litre (mmol), you can accurately tell whether you're in ketosis or not. These values can be measured by a doctor or with a blood ketone meter.

- For nutritional ketosis mmol levels range from 0.5 to 1.0
- For optimal ketosis mmol levels range 1.5 to 3.0

Mental clarity, sustained energy, reduced cravings, and proper blood sugar levels are also positive signs of ketosis. Be careful when you're trying to add back more carbs to your diet; add only a very small number each week and check that your body is still running on fat as its main source of energy!

## A note on macronutrients

The recipes you will find in this book include calorie and macro numbers. All calculations for these recipes have been done based on local ingredients. Ingredients around the world are generally the same, but different sources and manufacturing processes can result in slightly different nutrients present in your local ingredient. Do not worry about your local ingredients not meeting the ketogenic standards, but double checking from time to time doesn't hurt.

# Epilepsy and Ketosis

Characterized by seizures, epilepsy is a neurological condition that can be difficult to diagnose because it has various causes that can be difficult to separate and identify. In addition, it can involve a range of case-dependent symptoms including:

- Seizures
- Stiffening of all muscles
- Loss of muscle control
- Repetitive jerking muscle movements
- Temporary loss of awareness
- Sensory disturbances and mood swings

Some typical causes of epilepsy are birth defects, brain tumors, brain injuries, or strokes. Roughly 1% of the world's population has epilepsy – around 65 million individuals – with 80% of the cases occurring in developing countries.

There are several treatment options available. Perhaps the most serious one is brain surgery, which is a very physically invasive and frightening process. This used to be a last resort but in more recently the procedure has become safer and more effective.

On the milder end of the treatment scale, diets have been applied to prevent seizures and have shown mixed results. One such diet is the ketogenic diet, which has been shown to be quite useful for the prevention of seizures, even though the mechanisms that cause the effects are unknown. Some research has explored the neuron-protecting effects of the ketogenic diet.[28].

## Alcohol on a Ketogenic Vegan Diet

Alcoholic drinks are often high in carbohydrates, so limiting your alcohol intake is advisable. Since alcohol is metabolized in the liver, where ketones are produced by the metabolism, it is possible for increased alcohol consumption to cause an increased output of ketone bodies.

If you follow a ketogenic diet, you could therefore experience an increased "buzz" when consuming alcohol. Hangovers can also be intensified, and carb cravings may occur after alcohol intake. If you do have a drink, choose a hard liquor such as whiskey, rum, vodka, gin, or tequila. Avoid sugary alcoholic beverages like cocktails, and drink water along with the alcohol to mitigate its effects.

# Allergen Substitutes and Index

Following a vegan keto diet with a food allergy or sensitivity can be challenging—but not impossible. Below are some keto-proof substitutes for people with nut, soy, or peanut allergies.

## Tree nuts:

If you're allergic to one or more tree nuts, substitute seeds (or seed products like sunflower butter) for the nuts you need to avoid. Note that the taste will be quite different but the nutritional value is roughly the same.

For example, almond milk is an excellent plant-based milk because the unsweetened version contains zero grams net carbs. In case of a nut allergy, almond milk can be replaced with hemp milk, a cup (250 ml) of which only contains 0.7 grams net carbs. Unsweetened soy milk is another keto-friendly alternative.

## Peanuts:

Hemp, linseed, and flax seeds have a different taste but are options worth considering as a substitute for peanuts. When it comes to peanut butter, almond butter, cashew butter, sunflower seed butter, tahini, and pumpkin seed butter are great options that are all keto-proof!

## Soy:

Coconut aminos can be used as a substitute for soy sauce. If you also have a gluten intolerance, opt for tamari. Soy protein can be replaced with another low-carb (vegan) protein powder. Apart from soy, protein sources such as pea, rice, and hemp are also used to produce low-carb, vegan protein powders.

When it comes to tofu and tempeh, finding replacement can be challenging since beans and legumes are not keto-proof. Mushrooms are a decent substitute, but do not provide the high number of proteins found in tofu and other soy products. Seitan that is produced without soy is an option but contains a large amount of gluten. Make sure that seitan fits with the taste profile of the dish. For most savory meals, it's a fine choice.

## Allergy Index

Recipes with the ⓝ tag contain almonds, cashews, macadamia nuts, pecans, pistachios, or hazelnuts. The ⓢ tag indicates the use of soy beans or soy products like soy protein powder and tofu. A ⓟ tag indicates that peanuts or peanut-products are included in the ingredients.

# 1. Flax Egg

**Nutrition Information**
(per serving)
- Calories: 37 kcal
- Net Carbs: 0.2 g.
- Fat: 2.7 g.
- Protein: 1.1 g.
- Fiber: 1.9 g.
- Sugar: 0 g.

## INGREDIENTS:
- 1 tbsp. ground flaxseed
- 2-3 tbsp. lukewarm water

Total number of ingredients: 2

## METHOD:

1. Mix the ground flaxseed and water in a small bowl by using a spoon.
2. Cover the mixture and let it sit for 10 minutes.
3. Use the flax egg immediately, or, store it in an air-tight container in the fridge and consume within 5 days.

*Tip: You can use this mixture to replace a single egg in any recipe.*

## ESSENTIAL RECIPES

# 2. Simple Marinara Sauce

Serves: 8 | Prep Time: ~20 min |

**Nutrition Information**
(per serving)
- Calories: 23 kcal
- Net Carbs: 2.8 g.
- Fat: 1.1 g.
- Protein: 0.7 g.
- Fiber: 0.9 g.
- Sugar: 0.1 g.

## INGREDIENTS:
- 3 tbsp. olive oil
- 1 14-oz. can peeled tomatoes
  (no sugar added)
- ⅓ cup red onion (diced)
- 2 garlic cloves (minced)
- 2 tbsp. oregano (fresh and chopped,
  or 1 tbsp. dried)
- ½ tsp. cayenne pepper
- Salt and ground black pepper to taste
- Optional: 1 tbsp. sunflower seed butter

Total number of ingredients: 9

## METHOD:

1. Heat the olive oil in a medium-sized skillet over medium heat.
2. Add the onions, garlic, salt, and cayenne pepper. Sauté the onions until translucent while stirring the ingredients.
3. Add the peeled tomatoes and more salt and pepper to taste.
4. Stir the ingredients, cover the skillet, and allow the sauce to softly cook for 10 minutes.
5. Add the oregano, and if desired, stir in the optional butter.
6. Take the skillet off the heat. The sauce is now ready to be used in a recipe!
7. Alternatively, store the sauce in an airtight container in the fridge and consume within 3 days. Store for a maximum of 30 days in the freezer and thaw at room temperature.

*Tip: Use fresh herbs. Add a handful of chopped basil, parsley, or thyme for more flavor!*

# 3. Vegetable Broth

Serves: 10 | Prep Time: ~180 minutes |

**Nutrition Information**
(per serving)
- Calories: 0 kcal
- Net Carbs: 0 g.
- Fat: 0 g
- Protein: 0 g.
- Fiber: 0 g.
- Sugar: 0 g.

## INGREDIENTS:
- 4 onions (chopped)
- 4 cloves garlic (minced)
- 6 carrots (chopped)
- 5 celery stalks (leafless, chopped)
- 2 sweet potatoes (cubed)
- 2 bell peppers (red or yellow, seeded)
- 2 cups kale (chopped)
- 16 cups water
- 1 cup parsley (fresh)
- Salt and black pepper to taste
- Optional: 1 tbsp. red miso
- Optional: 2 tbsp. nutritional yeast

Total number of ingredients: 13

## METHOD

1. Preheat oven at 400°F/200°C and line a baking sheet with parchment paper.
2. Put the chopped onions, garlic, carrots, celery, sweet potato, bell peppers, kale and parsley on the baking sheet.
3. Drizzle the vegetables with a generous amount of olive oil, toss the vegetables around to coat evenly and put them in the oven.
4. Let the vegetables roast for about 1 hour or until they have browned.
5. Put a large pot over medium heat and add 16 cups of water.
6. While the water heats up, add the vegetables and turn the heat down to a simmer once it starts boiling.
7. Add the miso paste, parsley nutritional yeast and stir to make sure the miso paste is fully incorporated.
8. Let the broth simmer until the water has halved.
9. Add salt, pepper and any other desired spices to taste while stirring occasionally.
10. Take the pot off the stove and let the vegetable broth cool down for about 5 minutes.
11. Pour the broth through a sieve and collect it in a second large pot.
12. The leftover vegetables can be used as a delicious side dish.
13. Use the broth for a recipe or store it in batches in airtight containers in the fridge. Use or consume within 4 days. Store each batch individually in the freezer for a maximum of 30 days. Use a microwave or pot to defrost and reheat the broth.

# 4. Peanut Butter

Serves: 2 cups of peanut butter / 10 servings
| Prep Time: ~5 minutes |

**Nutrition Information**
(per serving)
- Calories: 134 kcal
- Net Carbs: 2.4 g.
- Fat: 11.2 g.
- Protein: 5.6 g.
- Fiber: 1.6 g.
- Sugar: 0.8 g.

## INGREDIENTS:
- 2 cups raw peanuts (unsalted)
- ½ tsp. Himalayan salt

Total number of ingredients: 2

## METHOD:

1. Preheat the oven to 375°F/190°C.
2. Put he peanuts on a baking sheet lined with parchment paper and roast them for about 10 minutes.
3. Transfer the peanuts to blender or food processor, blend for a minute, add the sea salt, and continue until the desired consistency is reached.
4. For the best flavor, chill the peanut butter before serving.

# 5. Chili Garlic Paste

Serves: 12 | Prep Time: ~5 minutes |

**Nutrition Information**
(per serving)
- Calories: 111 kcal
- Net Carbs: 2.64 g.
- Fat: 10.57 g.
- Protein: 1 g.
- Fiber: 2 g.
- Sugar: 0.75 g.

## INGREDIENTS:
- ½ cup MCT oil
- 1 cup green chili flakes
- 8 garlic cloves (minced)
- 1 tsp. salt
- Optional: 2 tsp. sugar
- Optional: ¼ cup Szechuan peppercorns

Total number of ingredients: 6

## METHOD:

1. Put all ingredients in a blender or food processor and pulse until smooth.
2. Store the chili garlic paste in a small, airtight container or mason jar in the fridge. Consume within 14 days. Store in the freezer for a maximum of 90 days and thaw at room temperature before serving.

*Tip: Chili garlic paste can be used as a marinade for tofu and tempeh or as mix it with nut and seed butters for delicious variations.*

# 6. Guacamole

Serves: 8 | Prep Time: ~15 min |

**Nutrition Information**
(per serving)
- Calories: 83 kcal
- Net Carbs: 2 g.
- Fat: 7.55 g.
- Protein: 1 g.
- Fiber: 4.1 g.
- Sugar: 1.2 g.

## INGREDIENTS:
- 3 medium avocados
  (peeled, pitted, halved)
- Juice of 1 lemon
- ⅓ cup red onion (minced)
- 1 garlic clove (minced)
- 1 handful fresh cilantro (chopped)
- Pinch of salt
- Black pepper to taste

Total number of ingredients: 7

## METHOD:

1. Put all ingredients in a blender or food processor and pulse until smooth. Alternatively, for a chunkier result, mash the ingredients in a medium-sized bowl with a fork.
2. Serve and enjoy!
3. Store the guacamole in an airtight container in the fridge and consume within 2 days. The guacamole can also be stored in the freezer for a maximum of 90 days. Thaw at room temperature before serving.

# 7. Mexican Salsa

**Nutrition Information**
(per serving)
- Calories: 30 kcal.
- Net Carbs: 4 g.
- Fat: 0.3 g.
- Protein: 0.8 g.
- Fiber: 2.1 g.
- Sugar: 4 g.

## INGREDIENTS:
- 4 large, firm tomatoes
- 1 fresh jalapeno
- ½ medium red onion
- 2 tbsp. fresh cilantro (chopped)
- 1 lime
- Salt & black pepper to taste

Total number of ingredients: 6

## METHOD:

1. Halve the jalapeno; remove and discard the stem, seeds, and placenta.
2. Add all the ingredients except the lime to a blender and blend for 30 seconds.
3. Transfer the sauce to a bowl and juice the lime on top of the sauce.
4. Give it a good stir and season to taste with salt and black pepper.
5. Let the sauce sit for 1 hour before serving and enjoy!
6. Alternatively, store the Mexican salsa in a small, airtight container or mason jar in the fridge. Consume within 4 days. Store in the freezer for a maximum of 60 days and thaw at room temperature before serving.

# 1. Chia Pudding with Blueberries

**Nutrition Information**
(per serving)
- Calories: 256 kcal
- Net Carbs: 6.2 g.
- Fat: 19.8. g
- Protein: 9.6 g.
- Fiber: 21.9 g.
- Sugar: 1.8 g.

## INGREDIENTS:
- 12 tbsp. chia seeds
- 3 cups unsweetened almond milk
- 1 cup water
- 4-6 drops stevia sweetener
- ¼ cup blueberries

Total number of ingredients: 5

## METHOD:

1. Put all the ingredients in a medium-sized bowl and stir. Alternatively, put all ingredients in a mason jar, close tightly, and shake.
2. Allow the pudding to sit for 5 minutes, then give it another stir (or shake).
3. Transfer the bowl or mason jar to the fridge. Refrigerate the pudding for at least 1 hour.
4. Give the pudding another stir, top it with the blueberries, and then serve and enjoy!
5. Alternatively, store the pudding in an airtight container in the fridge and consume within 4 days. Store for a maximum of 30 days in the freezer and thaw at room temperature.

*Note: This chia seed pudding is a great breakfast dish and can be prepared the night before serving. Simply allow the pudding to refrigerate overnight.*

*Tip: Mix up the combination of berries. Any low-carb fruit, like raspberries or strawberries, can be used as an addition to or substitute for blueberries!*

## BREAKFASTS

# 2. Coconut Porridge ⊛

**Nutrition Information**
(per serving)
- Calories: 251 kcal
- Net Carbs: 4.3 g.
- Fat: 22 g.
- Protein: 7.1 g.
- Fiber: 11 g.
- Sugar: 2 g.

## INGREDIENTS:
- ¼ cup dried coconut (unsweetened)
- ½ cup coconut milk (unsweetened)
- ⅔ cup water (or more depending on consistency)
- 3 tbsp. coconut flour
- 2 tbsp. psyllium husk
- ¼ tsp. vanilla extract
- 3-6 drops stevia sweetener (or more depending on the desired sweetness)
- Pinch of cinnamon
- Pinch of nutmeg
- 4 tbsp. toasted almond flakes
- Optional: pinch of salt

Total number of ingredients: 11

## METHOD:

1. Put a medium-sized pot over medium-high heat.
2. Toast the dried coconut in the pot while stirring for about 2 minutes.
3. Stir in the water and coconut milk.
4. Cover the pot and bring the mixture to a boil. Continue to stir in the remaining ingredients except the almond flakes.
5. Remove the pot from the heat and transfer the porridge to medium-sized bowls.
6. Top it with the almond flakes, some additional cinnamon, and enjoy!
7. Alternatively, store the porridge in an airtight container in the fridge and consume within 4 days. Store for a maximum of 60 days in the freezer and thaw at room temperature.

*Note: Substitute the vanilla extract and sweetener with a scoop of vanilla flavored organic soy protein powder. This will add protein and make the dish even more ketogenic-proof!*

*Tip: This dish can also be prepared in an instant pot. Simply add the ingredients—except the almond flakes—and set the pot to cook the porridge right before waking up!*

# 3. Protein Nut 'N Seed Bread

Serves: 10 | Prep Time: ~60 min |

**Nutrition Information**
(per serving)
- Calories: 393 kcal
- Net Carbs: 4.3 g.
- Fat: 35.2 g.
- Protein: 13.8 g.
- Fiber: 6.6 g.
- Sugar: 1.7 g.

## INGREDIENTS:
- ¼ cup almonds
- ¼ cup hazelnuts
- ½ cup pumpkin seeds
- ¼ cup flax seeds
- 3 flax eggs (page 27)
- 3 tbsp. sesame seeds
- 3 cups almond flour
- 1 scoop organic soy protein powder (unflavored; or alternatively, use vanilla flavor)
- 2 tbsp. coconut flour
- 1½ tsp. baking soda
- Pinch of salt
- ½ cup unsweetened almond milk
- 1 tbsp. apple cider vinegar
- ⅓ cup coconut oil
- 2 tbsp. low-carb maple syrup
- 2 tbsp. water (or more depending on dough consistency)

Total number of ingredients: 16

## METHOD:
1. Preheat the oven to 350°F/180°C.
2. Line a loaf pan with parchment paper.
3. Put the almonds and hazelnuts in a blender or food processor. Pulse until ground.
4. Add the seeds and blend the ingredients again until ground. Scrape the sides of the blender or food processor if necessary.
5. Transfer the mixture to a large bowl and mix in the almond flour, baking soda, and salt with a whisk or spoon.
6. Take a separate medium-sized bowl and add the almond milk, protein powder, flax eggs, coconut oil, maple syrup, and vinegar. Stir well until all the ingredients are incorporated. Add 2 tablespoons of water (or more, if necessary), and stir.
7. Allow the wet mixture to sit for a few minutes. Stir again and then add it to the dry mixture in the large bowl.
8. Use a whisk or spoon to combine all ingredients.
9. Transfer the dough to the loaf pan lined with parchment paper.
10. Put the loaf pan in the oven and bake the bread for 50 minutes or until a fork comes out clean. Take the loaf pan out of the oven and allow the bread to cool down.
11. Remove the parchment paper, transfer the bread to a cutting board, and slice it into 10 slices before serving. Enjoy!
12. Alternatively, store the bread in an airtight container in the fridge and consume within 5 days. Store for a maximum of 60 days in the freezer and thaw at room temperature.

*Note: You can substitute almonds for hazelnuts and vice versa. You can also substitute hazelnut flour for the almond flour, or use a mixture of both.*

*Tip: Add more seeds and crushed nuts on top of the dough. Use a protein powder with little-to-no flavor. Serve this bread with Avocado and Cauliflower Hummus (page 53)!*

# 1. Nutty Protein Shake

**Nutrition Information**
(per serving)
- Calories: 618 kcal
- Net Carbs: 4.4 g.
- Fat: 51.3 g.
- Protein: 34 g.
- Fiber: 4.9 g.
- Sugar: 3 g.

## INGREDIENTS:
- 2 tbsp. coconut oil
- 2 cups unsweetened almond milk
- 2 tbsp. peanut butter (page 30)
- 1 scoop organic soy protein powder (chocolate flavor)
- 2-4 ice cubes
- 4-6 drops stevia sweetener
- Optional: 1 tsp. vegan creamer
- Optional: 1 tsp. cocoa powder

Total number of ingredients: 8

## METHOD:

1. Add all the above listed ingredients—except the optional ingredients—to a blender, and blend for 2 minutes.
2. Transfer the shake to a large cup or shaker. If desired, top the shake with the optional vegan creamer and/or cocoa powder.
3. Stir before serving and enjoy!
4. Alternatively, store the smoothie in an airtight container or a mason jar, keep it in the fridge, and consume within 3 days. Store for a maximum of 30 days in the freezer and thaw at room temperature.

## SMOOTHIES

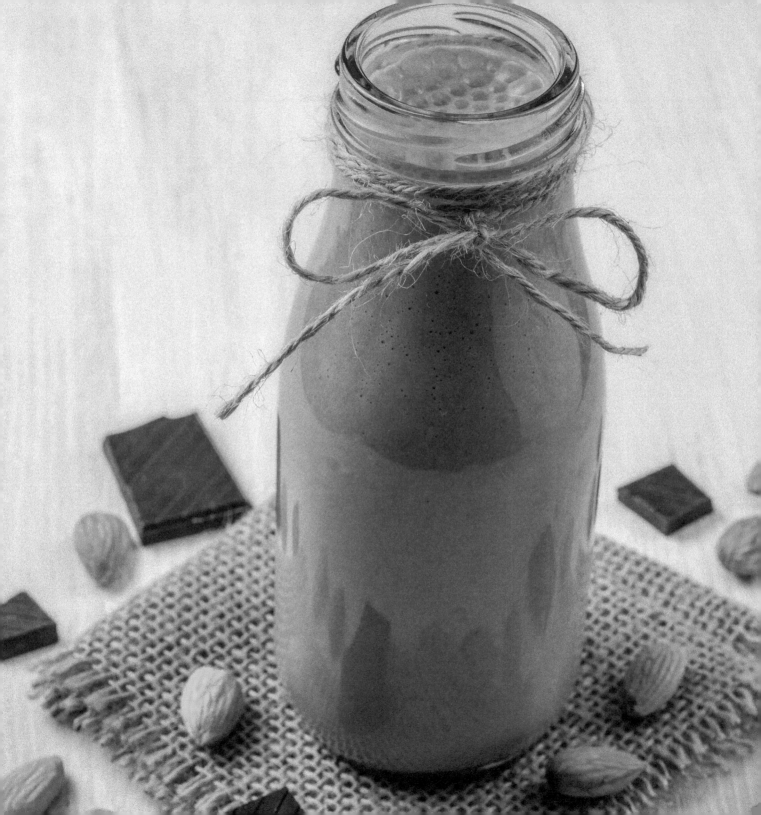

# 2. Chocolate-Vanilla Almond Milk

**Nutrition Information**
(per serving)
- Calories: 422 kcal
- Net Carbs: 1.3 g.
- Fat: 34.8 g.
- Protein: 25.5 g.
- Fiber: 2.7 g.
- Sugar: 0.8 g.

## INGREDIENTS:
- 2 tbsp. coconut oil
- 1½ cups unsweetened almond milk
- ½ vanilla stick (crushed)
- 1 scoop organic soy protein powder (chocolate flavor)
- 4-6 drops stevia sweetener
- Optional: ½ tsp. cinnamon
- Optional: 1-2 ice cubes

Total number of ingredients: 7

## METHOD:

1. Add all the listed ingredients to a blender—except the ice—but including the optional cinnamon if desired.
2. Blend the ingredients for 1 minute; then if desired, add the optional ice cubes and blend for another 30 seconds.
3. Transfer the milk to a large cup or shaker, top with some additional cinnamon, serve, and enjoy!
4. Alternatively, store the smoothie in an airtight container or a mason jar, keep it in the fridge, and consume within 3 days. Store for a maximum of 30 days in the freezer and thaw at room temperature.

# 3. Chia & Coco Shake

Serves: 1 | Prep Time: ~5 min |

**Nutrition Information**
(per serving)
- Calories: 593 kcal
- Net Carbs: 7.4 g.
- Fat: 45.6 g.
- Protein: 36 g.
- Fiber: 13.9 g.
- Sugar: 3 g.

## INGREDIENTS:
- 1 tbsp. chia seeds
- 6 tbsp. water
- 1 cup coconut milk
- 2 tbsp. peanut butter (page 30)
- 1 tbsp. MCT oil (or coconut oil)
- 1 scoop organic soy protein powder
  (chocolate flavor)
- Pinch of Himalayan salt
- 2-4 ice cubes or ½ cup of water

Total number of ingredients: 8

## METHOD:

1. Mix the chia seeds and 6 tablespoons of water in a small bowl; let sit for at least 30 minutes.
2. Transfer the soaked chia seeds and all other listed ingredients to a blender and blend for 2 minutes.
3. Transfer the shake to a large cup or shaker, serve, and enjoy!
4. Alternatively, store the smoothie in an airtight container or a mason jar, keep it in the fridge, and consume within 3 days. Store for a maximum of 30 days in the freezer and thaw at room temperature.

*Note: This shake will supply you with some additional minerals and electrolytes found in the Himalayan salt!*

# 4. Raspberry Protein Shake ⑧

Serves: 1 | Prep Time: ~5 min |

**Nutrition Information**
(per serving)
- Calories: 311 kcal
- Net Carbs: 6.9 g.
- Fat: 19.3 g.
- Protein: 26.8 g.
- Fiber: 5 g.
- Sugar: 4.8 g.

## INGREDIENTS:

- 1 cup full-fat coconut milk (or alternatively, use almond milk)
- Optional: ¼ cup coconut cream
- 1 scoop organic soy protein (chocolate or vanilla flavor)
- ½ cup raspberries (fresh or frozen)
- 1 tbsp. low-carb maple syrup
- Optional: 2-4 ice cubes

Total number of ingredients: 6

## METHOD:

1. Add all the ingredients to a blender, including the optional coconut cream and ice cubes if desired, and blend for 1 minute.
2. Transfer the shake to a large cup or shaker, and enjoy!
3. Alternatively, store the smoothie in an airtight container or a mason jar, keep it in the fridge, and consume within 2 days. Store for a maximum of 30 days in the freezer and thaw at room temperature.

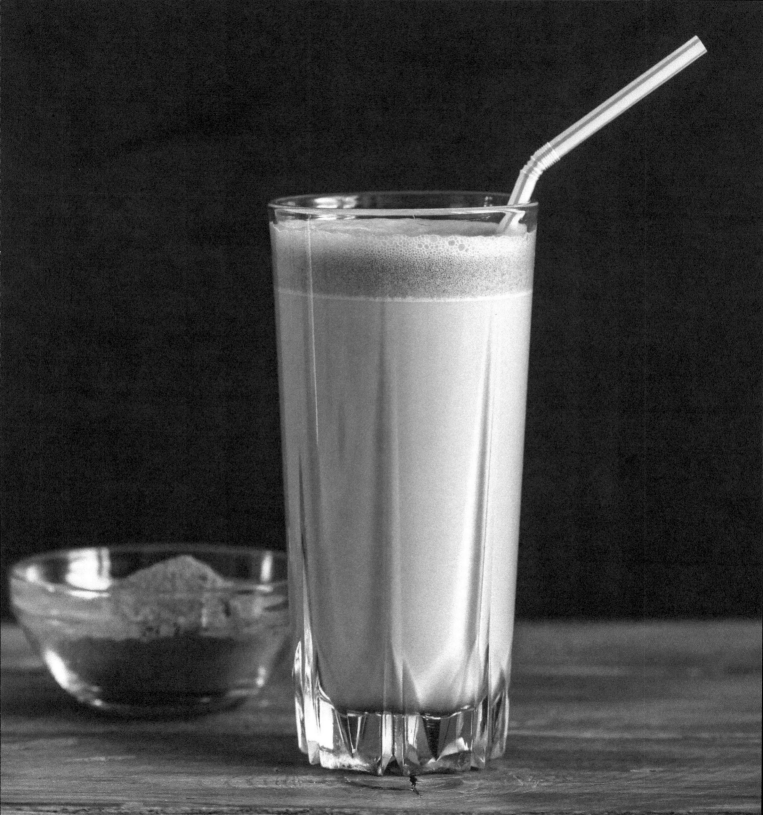

# 5. Fat-Rich Protein Espresso

Serves: 1 | Prep Time: ~5 min |

**Nutrition Information**
(per serving)
- Calories: 441 kcal
- Net Carbs: 5.6 g.
- Fat: 34.8 g.
- Protein: 25.4 g.
- Fiber: 6.9 g.
- Sugar: 2.8 g.

## INGREDIENTS:
- 1 cup espresso (freshly brewed)
- 2 tbsp. coconut butter (or alternatively, use coconut oil)
- 1 scoop organic soy protein (chocolate flavor)
- ½ vanilla stick
- 4 ice cubes or ½ cup boiled water
- Optional: 1 tbsp. cocoa powder
- Optional: ½ tsp. cinnamon
- 2 tbsp. coconut cream

Total number of ingredients: 8

## METHOD:

1. Make sure to use fresh, hot espresso.
2. Add all the listed ingredients to a heat-safe blender, including the ice or boiled water and optional ingredients (if desired). Use ice to make iced espresso, or hot water for a warm treat.
3. Blend the ingredients for 1 minute and transfer to a large coffee cup.
4. Top the coffee with the coconut cream, stir, serve and enjoy!
5. Alternatively, store the smoothie in an airtight container or a mason jar, keep it in the fridge, and consume within 3 days. Store for a maximum of 30 days in the freezer and thaw at room temperature.

# 6. Forest Fruit Blaster ⑨

**Nutrition Information**
(per serving)
- Calories: 603 kcal
- Net Carbs: 11.5 g.
- Fat: 38.1 g.
- Protein: 52.9 g.
- Fiber: 4.5 g.
- Sugar: 9.9 g.

## INGREDIENTS:
- ¼ cup mixed berries (fresh or frozen)
- ½ kiwi (peeled)
- 2 cups full-fat coconut milk
- 2 scoops organic soy protein (vanilla flavor)
- ½ cup water
- Optional: 2 ice cubes

Total number of ingredients: 6

## METHOD:

1. Add all the ingredients to a blender, including the optional ice if desired, and blend for 1 minute.
2. Transfer the shake to a large cup or shaker and enjoy!
3. Alternatively, store the smoothie in an airtight container or a mason jar, keep it in the fridge, and consume within 2 days. Store for a maximum of 30 days in the freezer and thaw at room temperature.

# 7. Vanilla Milkshake 🍼 🥥

Serves: 1 | Prep Time: ~5 min |

**Nutrition Information**
(per serving)
- Calories: 600 kcal
- Net Carbs: 5.3 g.
- Fat: 46.6 g.
- Protein: 39.3 g.
- Fiber: 4.3 g.
- Sugar: 3.3 g.

## INGREDIENTS:
- 2 tbsp. cocoa butter
- 2 cups unsweetened almond milk
- ¼ cup hemp seeds
- 2 tbsp. coconut whipped cream
- 4-6 drops stevia sweetener
- 1 scoop organic soy protein (vanilla flavor)
- 4 ice cubes

Total number of ingredients: 7

## METHOD:

1. Add all the ingredients—except the coconut whipped cream—to a blender and blend for 2 minutes.
2. Transfer the shake to a large cup or shaker.
3. Serve with the coconut whipped cream on top, stir, and enjoy!
4. Alternatively, store the smoothie in an airtight container or a mason jar, keep it in the fridge, and consume within 3 days. Store for a maximum of 30 days in the freezer and thaw at room temperature.

# 8. Raspberry Lemon Protein Smoothie

Serves: 2 | Prep Time: ~5 min |

**Nutrition Information**
(per serving)
- Calories: 314 kcal
- Net Carbs: 6.7 g.
- Fat: 23.7 g.
- Protein: 17.8 g.
- Fiber: 6.3 g.
- Sugar: 4.2 g.

## INGREDIENTS:
- ¼ cup flaxseeds
- ½ cup water
- 2 cups full-fat coconut milk
- 1 organic lemon (with peel)
- ½ cup raspberries (fresh or frozen)
- 1 scoop organic soy protein (vanilla flavor)
- 4-6 drops stevia sweetener
- 2 ice cubes

Total number of ingredients: 8

## METHOD:

1. Mix the flaxseeds with the water in a medium-sized bowl. Allow the mixture to sit for up to 30 minutes.
2. Add the soaked flaxseeds and the other ingredients to a blender and blend for 2 minutes.
3. Transfer the smoothie to a large cup or shaker, and enjoy!
4. Alternatively, store the smoothie in an airtight container or a mason jar, keep it in the fridge, and consume within 3 days. Store for a maximum of 30 days in the freezer and thaw at room temperature.

# 9. Breakfast Booster ⊛

Serves: 1 | Prep Time: ~5 min |

**Nutrition Information**
(per serving)
- Calories: 357 kcal
- Net Carbs: 5.8 g.
- Fat: 25.8 g.
- Protein: 24.8 g.
- Fiber: 4.7 g.
- Sugar: 3.2 g.

## INGREDIENTS:
- 1 cup coconut milk
- 2 tbsp. cocoa butter
- 1 scoop organic soy protein (vanilla flavor)
- 4 ice cubes
- Pinch of Himalayan salt
- 5 strawberries (fresh or frozen)
- 1 tsp. matcha powder
- 1 tsp. guarana powder
- 4-6 drops stevia sweetener

Total number of ingredients: 9

## METHOD:

1. Add all the required ingredients to a blender and blend for 1 minute.
2. Transfer the shake to a large cup or shaker, and enjoy!
3. Alternatively, store the smoothie in an airtight container or a mason jar, keep it in the fridge, and consume within 2 days. Store for a maximum of 30 days in the freezer and thaw at room temperature.

# 10. Cinnamon Pear Protein Shake

**Nutrition Information**
(per serving)
- Calories: 398 kcal
- Net Carbs: 5.4 g.
- Fat: 28 g.
- Protein: 28.8 g.
- Fiber: 14.9 g.
- Sugar: 4.4 g.

## INGREDIENTS:
- 1 tsp. freeze-dried pear powder
- 1 medium Hass avocado
  (peeled, pitted, and halved)
- 2 cups unsweetened almond milk
- 1 scoop organic soy protein
  (vanilla flavor)
- ½ tsp. cinnamon
- 4-6 drops stevia sweetener
- 2 ice cubes

Total number of ingredients: 7

## METHOD:

1. Add all the required ingredients to a blender, including the optional ice cubes if desired, and blend for 1 minute.
2. Transfer to a large cup or shaker and enjoy!
3. Alternatively, store the smoothie in an airtight container or a mason jar, keep it in the fridge, and consume within 3 days. Store for a maximum of 30 days in the freezer and thaw at room temperature.

# 11. Raspberry Coco Shake

**Serves: 1 | Prep Time: ~5 min |**

**Nutrition Information**
(per serving)
- Calories: 383 kcal
- Net Carbs: 5.6 g.
- Fat: 28.6 g.
- Protein: 24.6 g.
- Fiber: 6.5 g.
- Sugar: 4.8 g.

## INGREDIENTS:
- 1 ½ cups unsweetened almond milk
- 1 scoop organic soy protein (chocolate flavor)
- ½ cup full-fat coconut milk
- ½ cup raspberries (fresh or frozen)
- 4 drops stevia sweetener
- 2 ice cubes

Total number of ingredients: 6

## METHOD:

1. Put all the ingredients in a blender and blend for about 1 minute, or until the shake reaches the desired consistency.
2. Transfer the shake to a large cup or shaker and enjoy!
3. Alternatively, store the smoothie in an airtight container or mason jar in the fridge, and consume within 3 days. Store for a maximum of 30 days in the freezer and thaw at room temperature before serving.

*Tip: Use more or fewer ice cubes, depending on the desired consistency.*

# 12. Bulletproof Protein Shake ⑧

**Nutrition Information**
(per serving)
- Calories: 448 kcal
- Net Carbs: 5 g.
- Fat: 39.55 g.
- Protein: 16 g.
- Fiber: 12.7 g.
- Sugar: 4.5 g.

## INGREDIENTS:
- 4 tbsp. chia seeds
- ½ cup water
- 1 medium Hass avocado (pitted, peeled)
- 1 scoop organic soy protein (chocolate flavor)
- 1 cup full-fat coconut milk
- 2 tsp. vanilla extract
- Pinch of Himalayan salt
- 4 ice cubes

Total number of ingredients: 8

## METHOD:

1. Put the chia seeds and water in a blender and allow the seeds to soak at least 10 minutes.
2. Add all remaining ingredients to the blender and blend for about 1 minute, or until the shake reaches the desired consistency.
3. Transfer the shake to two large cups or shakers and enjoy!
4. Alternatively, store the smoothie in an airtight container or canning jar in the fridge, and consume within 2 days. Store for a maximum of 30 days in the freezer and thaw at room temperature before serving.

*Tip: Use more or fewer ice cubes, depending on the desired consistency.*

# 1. Raw Zoodles with Avocado 'N Nuts

Serves: 2 | Prep Time: ~10 min |

**Nutrition Information**
(per serving)
- Calories: 317 kcal
- Net Carbs: 7.4 g.
- Fat: 28.1 g.
- Protein: 7.2 g.
- Fiber: 8.9 g.
- Sugar: 5.6 g.

## INGREDIENTS:
- 1 medium zucchini (spiralized into zoodles or sliced into very thin slices)
- 1½ cups basil
- ⅓ cup water
- 5 tbsp. pine nuts
- 2 tbsp. lemon juice
- 1 medium avocado (peeled, pitted, and sliced)
- Optional: 2 tbsp. olive oil
- 6 yellow cherry tomatoes (halved)
- Optional: 6 red cherry tomatoes (halved)
- Sea salt and black pepper to taste

Total number of ingredients: 11

## METHOD:

1. Add the basil, water, nuts, lemon juice, avocado slices, optional olive oil (if desired), salt, and pepper to a blender.
2. Blend the ingredients into a smooth mixture. Add more salt and pepper to taste and blend again.
3. Divide the sauce and the zucchini noodles between two medium-sized bowls for serving, and combine in each.
4. Top the mixtures with the halved yellow cherry tomatoes, and the optional red cherry tomatoes (if desired); serve and enjoy!
5. Alternatively, store the zoodles in the fridge using an airtight container and consume within 2 days.

*Tip: Add more spiralized or sliced veggies—like cabbage—to add flavor. The salad can be topped with additional nuts, seeds, or more oil.*

## LUNCHES

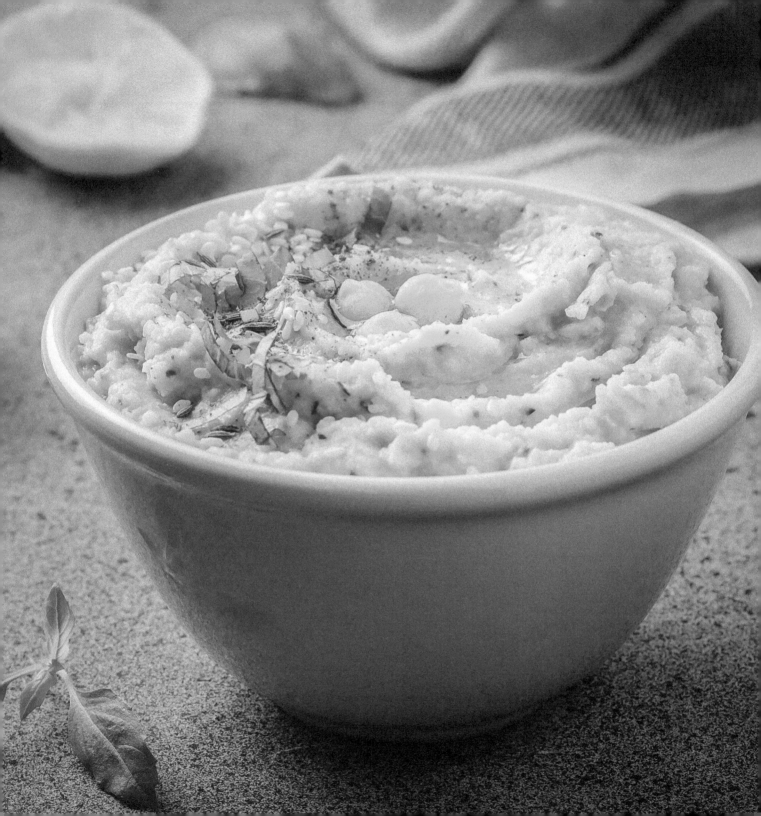

# 2. Avocado and Cauliflower Hummus

Serves: 2 | Prep Time: ~20 min |

**Nutrition Information**
(per serving)
- Calories: 416 kcal
- Net Carbs: 8.4 g.
- Fat: 40.3 g.
- Protein: 3.3 g.
- Fiber: 10.3 g.
- Sugar: 7.1 g.

## INGREDIENTS:
- 1 medium cauliflower
  (stem removed and chopped)
- 1 large Hass avocado
  (peeled, pitted, and chopped)
- ¼ cup extra virgin olive oil
- 2 garlic cloves
- ½ tbsp. lemon juice
- ½ tsp. onion powder
- Sea salt and ground black pepper to taste
- 2 large carrots (peeled and cut into fries,
  or use store-bought raw carrot fries)
- Optional: ¼ cup fresh cilantro (chopped)

Total number of ingredients: 10

## METHOD:

1. Preheat the oven to 450°F/220°C, and line a baking tray with aluminum foil.
2. Put the chopped cauliflower on the baking tray and drizzle with 2 tablespoons of olive oil.
3. Roast the chopped cauliflower in the oven for 20-25 minutes, until lightly brown.
4. Remove the tray from the oven and allow the cauliflower to cool down.
5. Add all the ingredients—except the carrots and optional fresh cilantro—to a food processor or blender, and blend the ingredients into a smooth hummus.
6. Transfer the hummus to a medium-sized bowl, cover, and put it in the fridge for at least 30 minutes.
7. Take the hummus out of the fridge and, if desired, top it with the optional chopped cilantro and more salt and pepper to taste; serve with the carrot fries, and enjoy!
8. Alternatively, store it in the fridge in an airtight container, and consume within 2 days.

*Tip: For baked fries, bake the carrot slices in the oven with olive oil, salt, and pepper at 450°F/220°C for 15-20 minutes. This hummus can also be served on top of Almond Bread (page 57).*

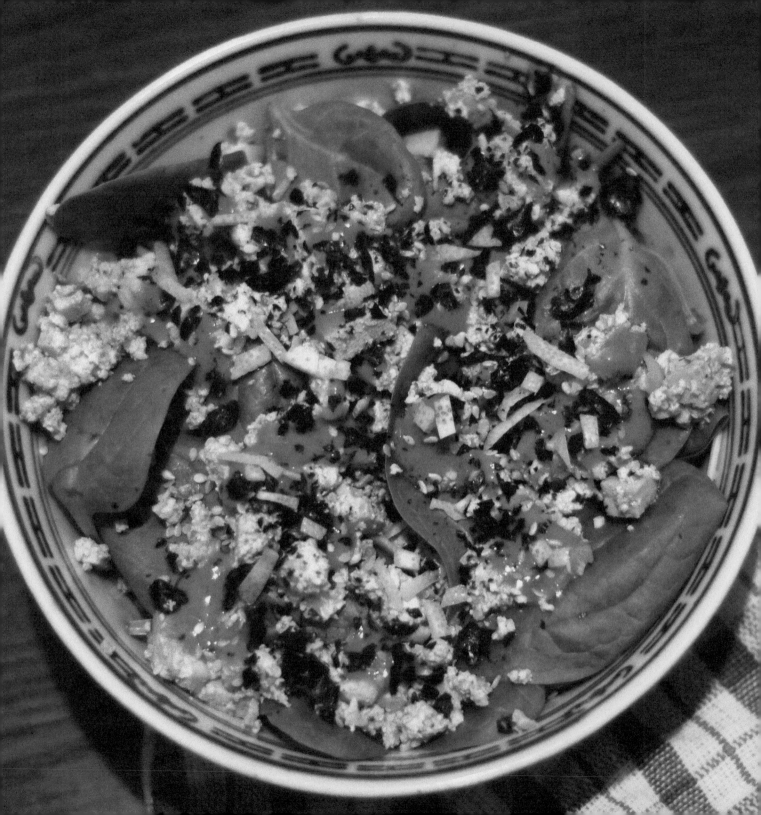

# 3. Spinach and mashed tofu salad

Serves: 4 | Prep Time: ~20 min |

**Nutrition Information**
(per serving)
- Calories: 166 kcal
- Net Carbs: 5.5 g.
- Fat: 10.7 g.
- Protein: 11.3 g.
- Fiber: 2.8 g.
- Sugar: 2.2 g.

## INGREDIENTS:
- 2 8-oz. blocks firm tofu (drained)
- 4 cups baby spinach leaves
- 4 tbsp. cashew butter
- 1½ tbsp. soy sauce
- 1-inch piece ginger (finely chopped)
- 1 tsp. red miso paste
- 2 tbsp. sesame seeds
- 1 tsp. organic orange zest
- 1 tsp. nori flakes
- Optional: 2 tbsp. water

Total number of ingredients: 10

## METHOD:

1. Use paper towels to absorb any excess water left in the tofu before crumbling both blocks into small pieces.
2. In a large bowl, combine the mashed tofu with the spinach leaves.
3. Mix the remaining ingredients in another small bowl and, if desired, add the optional water for a more smooth dressing.
4. Pour this dressing over the mashed tofu and spinach leaves.
5. Transfer the bowl to the fridge and allow the salad to chill for up to one hour. Doing so will guarantee a better flavor. Or, the salad can be served right away. Enjoy!
6. Alternatively, store the spinach and mashed tofu salad in the fridge using an airtight container. Consume within 2 days.

# 4. Cauliflower Sushi ⊚

Serves: 4 | Prep Time: ~30 min |

**Nutrition Information**
(per serving)
- Calories: 189 kcal
- Net Carbs: 7.6 g.
- Fat: 14.4 g.
- Protein: 6.1 g.
- Fiber: 7.45 g.
- Sugar: 6 g.

## INGREDIENTS:
*Sushi Base:*
- 6 cups cauliflower florets
  (or 15-oz. pack cauliflower rice)
- ½ cup vegan cheese
  (see mozzarella recipe)
- 1 medium spring onion (diced)
- 4 nori sheets
- Sea salt and pepper to taste
- 1 tbsp. rice vinegar or sushi vinegar
- Optional: 1 medium garlic clove (minced)

*Filling:*
- 1 medium Hass avocado (peeled, sliced)
- ½ medium cucumber (skinned, sliced)
- 4 asparagus spears
- Optional: handful of enoki mushrooms

Total number of ingredients: 12

## METHOD:

1. Put the cauliflower florets in a food processor or blender. Pulse the florets into a rice-like substance. When using readymade cauliflower rice, add this to the blender.
2. Add the vegan cheese, spring onions, and vinegar to the food processor or blender. Top these ingredients with salt and pepper to taste, and pulse everything into a chunky mixture. Make sure not to turn the ingredients into a puree by pulsing too long.
3. Taste and add more vinegar, salt, or pepper to taste. Add the optional minced garlic clove to the blender and pulse again for a few seconds.
4. Lay out the nori sheets and spread the cauliflower rice mixture out evenly between the sheets. Make sure to leave at least 2 inches of the top and bottom edges empty.
5. Place one or more combinations of multiple filling ingredients along the center of the spread out rice mixture. Experiment with different ingredients per nori sheet for the best flavor.
6. Roll up each nori sheet tightly. (Using a sushi mat will make this easier.)
7. Either serve the sushi as a nori roll, or, slice each roll up into sushi pieces.
8. Serve right away with a small amount of wasabi, pickled ginger, and soy sauce!
9. Alternatively, store the sushi in an airtight container in the fridge and consume within 3 days. Store the sushi in the freezer for a maximum of 60 days and thaw at room temperature.

*Tip: You can choose to add some mashed (boiled) egg or an omelet as an ingredient for the sushi filling. Doing so will make the dish ovo and adds protein.*

# 5. Keto Curry Almond Bread ⊚

Serves: 2 | Prep Time: ~30 min |

**Nutrition Information**
(per serving)
- Calories: 372 kcal
- Net Carbs: 5.1 g.
- Fat: 34.7 g.
- Protein: 8.3 g.
- Fiber: 9.5 g.
- Sugar: 2.2 g.

## INGREDIENTS:
- ½ cup almond flour (or coconut flour)
- ¼ cup almond milk
- ¼ cup ground flaxseed
- 2 tbsp. coconut oil
- 2 tbsp. red curry paste
- ½ tsp. salt
- ½ tsp. cane sugar (or stevia powder)
- 2 kaffir lime leaves (chopped)
- 2 tsp. dried ginger (or fresh, minced)
- Optional: ¼ cup water
- Optional: 4 tbsp. coconut flakes

Total number of ingredients: 12

## METHOD:

1. Line a baking sheet with parchment paper.
2. In a medium bowl, mix the almond milk with the sugar, salt, and ground flaxseeds. Stir well and let it sit for 10 minutes.
3. Add the flour, kaffir lime leaves, and ginger to the bowl.
4. Incorporate all ingredients using your hands or an electric mixer. Add some of the optional water to make the mixing easier.
5. Divide the dough into two pieces and flatten these out onto the baking sheet.
6. Grease both sides of the dough with the coconut oil and apply a tablespoon of red curry paste on the top side of each flattened bread.
7. Allow the pieces of bread to rest for an hour at room temperature.
8. Preheat the oven to 400°F / 200°C.
9. Bake the bread for about 15 minutes, until golden brown on top.
10. Top the breads with the optional coconut flakes.
11. Serve and enjoy!
12. Alternatively, store the breads at room temperature or in the fridge using an airtight container and consume within 1-2 days.

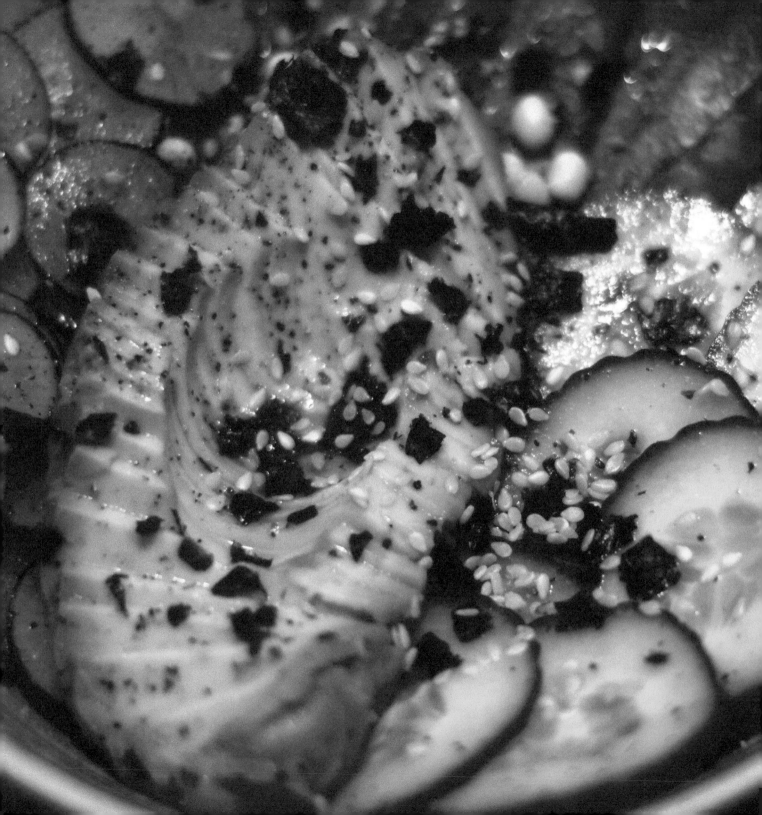

# 6. Cucumber Edamame Salad ⊛

Serves: 2 | Prep Time: ~40 min |

**Nutrition Information**
(per serving)
- Calories: 409 kcal
- Net Carbs: 7.1 g.
- Fat: 38.25 g.
- Protein: 7.6 g.
- Fiber: 9.2 g.
- Sugar: 3.95 g.

## INGREDIENTS:
- 3 tbsp. avocado oil
- 1 cup cucumber (sliced into thin rounds)
- ½ cup fresh sugar snap peas (sliced or whole)
- ½ cup fresh edamame
- ¼ cup radish (sliced)
- 1 large Hass avocado (peeled, pitted, sliced)
- 1 nori sheet (crumbled)
- 2 tsp. roasted sesame seeds
- 1 tsp. salt

Total number of ingredients: 9

## METHOD:

1. Bring a medium-sized pot filled half way with water to a boil over medium-high heat.
2. Add the sugar snaps and cook them for about 2 minutes.
3. Take the pot off the heat, drain the excess water, transfer the sugar snaps to a medium-sized bowl and set aside for now.
4. Fill the pot with water again, add the teaspoon of salt and bring to a boil over medium-high heat.
5. Add the edamame to the pot and let them cook for about 6 minutes.
6. Take the pot off the heat, drain the excess water, transfer the soybeans to the bowl with sugar snaps and let them cool down for about 5 minutes.
7. Combine all ingredients, except the nori crumbs and roasted sesame seeds, in a medium-sized bowl.
8. Carefully stir, using a spoon, until all ingredients are evenly coated in oil.
9. Top the salad with the nori crumbs and roasted sesame seeds.
10. Transfer the bowl to the fridge and allow the salad to cool for at least 30 minutes.
11. Serve chilled and enjoy!
12. Alternatively, store the cucumber edamame salad and the nori and sesame seeds in separate airtight containers in the fridge. Consume within 2 days. Store in the freezer for a maximum of 30 days and thaw at room temperature before serving.

# 7. Egg Roll Bowl ⑧

Serves: 2 | Prep Time: ~15 min |

**Nutrition Information**
(per serving)
- Calories: 269 kcal
- Net Carbs: 9.5 g.
- Fat: 17.6 g.
- Protein: 16.7 g.
- Fiber: 9.4 g.
- Sugar: 6.1 g.

## INGREDIENTS:
- 2 7-oz. packs shirataki noodles
- 1 tbsp. coconut oil
- 1 tbsp. sesame oil
- 1 tbsp. rice vinegar
- 1 12-oz. pack extra firm tofu (drained, cubed)
- 1 red onion (diced)
- 2 garlic cloves (minced)
- 1-inch fresh ginger (finely minced)
- 4 tbsp. low sodium soy sauce
- ½ cup red pickled cabbage (chopped)
- ½ cup carrots (matchsticks or julienned)

Total number of ingredients: 11

## METHOD:

1. In a medium bowl, rinse the shirataki noodles with cold water, drain, and set aside.
2. Take a large skillet and put it over medium-high heat.
3. Add the coconut oil and sesame oil to the skillet.
4. Add the rice vinegar, tofu cubes, and onions to the skillet. Stir-fry the ingredients until the onions start to caramelize.
5. Blend in the garlic, ginger, and soy sauce. Allow the ingredients to cook for a minute while occasionally stirring.
6. Add the carrots to the skillet and cook for another 5 minutes while stirring occasionally.
7. Take the skillet off the heat, divide the shirataki noodles over 2 medium bowls, top each portion with half of the tofu mixture and chopped cabbage, serve, and enjoy!
8. Alternatively, store the tofu mixture and noodles separated in the fridge. Use airtight containers and consume within 3 days. Store in the freezer for a maximum of 30 days and thaw at room temperature. Use a microwave, toaster oven or skillet to reheat the dish.

# 8. Shio Koji Karaage Tofu

**Nutrition Information**
(per serving)
- Calories: 355 kcal
- Net Carbs: 4.9 g.
- Fat: 32 g.
- Protein: 11.3 g.
- Fiber: 2.4 g.
- Sugar: 4.1 g.

## INGREDIENTS:
- Extra light olive oil (for deep-frying)
- 1 12-oz. pack extra firm tofu (drained, cubed)
- 4 tbsp. Hikari Shio Koji
- 1 tsp. fresh ginger (finely chopped)
- 1 garlic clove (minced)
- 2 tsp. soy sauce
- ½ cup almond flour
- Optional: lemon wedges

Total number of ingredients: 8

## METHOD:

1. In a large bowl or Ziploc bag, combine the tofu cubes with the Hikari Shio Koji, ginger, garlic, and soy sauce.
2. Use your hands to make sure the tofu is evenly coated. Cover the bowl or close the Ziploc bag and put in the fridge. Marinate the tofu for at least 30 minutes up to a maximum of 1 day.
3. Heat up a pot with enough of the olive oil to deep fry the tofu cubes. The ideal temperature for the oil is 325°F /160°F.
4. Take the tofu cubes out of the fridge and cover the cubes with almond flour. This can be done in the bowl or Ziploc bag. Use your hands to evenly coat all tofu cubes with flour.
5. Drop the coated cubes gently into the pot and fry until they're lightly browned.
6. When the tofu cubes are ready, transfer them to a plate lined with paper towels to drain the excess oil.
7. Serve the shio koji karaage tofu, garnished with the optional lemon wedges if desired, and enjoy!
8. Alternatively, store the dish in an airtight container in the fridge. Consume within 3 days. Store in the freezer for a maximum of 30 days, and thaw at room temperature. Use a toaster oven or skillet to reheat the shio koji karaage tofu.

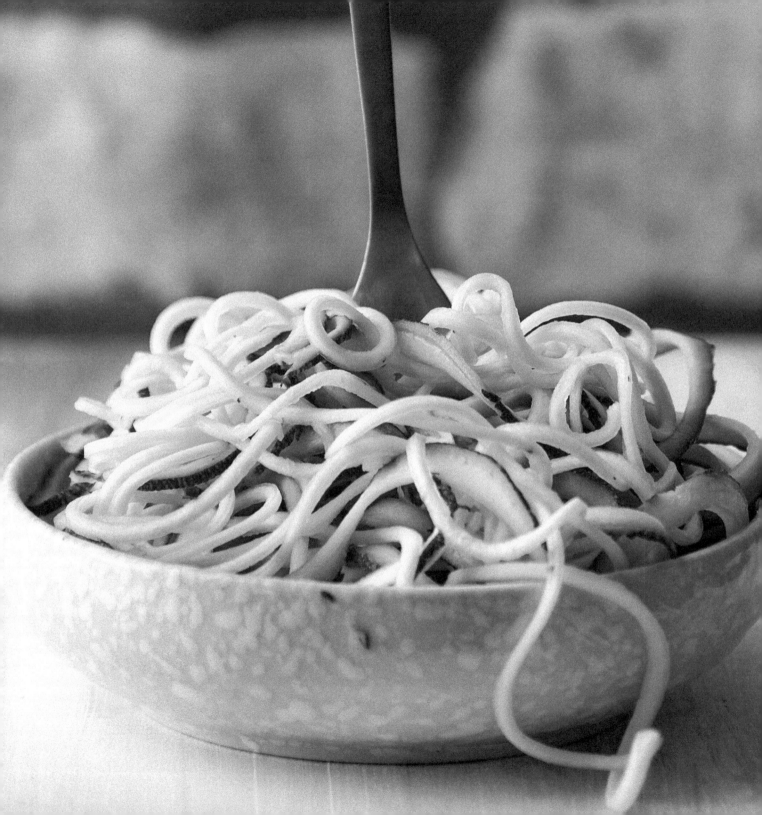

# 9. Zoodle Pesto Salad ⊛

Serves: 2 | Prep Time: ~20 min |

**Nutrition Information**
(per serving)
 - Calories: 389 kcal
 - Net Carbs: 6.5 g.
 - Fat: 37 g.
 - Protein: 5.9 g.
 - Fiber: 4.2 g.
 - Sugar: 5.5 g.

## INGREDIENTS:
 - 2 medium zucchinis (spiralized into zoodles or sliced lengthwise very thinly)
 - ¼ cup extra virgin olive oil
 - 1 ½ cups fresh baby spinach leaves
 - ¼ cup walnuts (crushed)
 - 1 tsp. garlic powder
 - Sea salt and ground black pepper to taste
 - ¼ cup capers (chopped)
 - Optional: ½ cup of vegan cheese (page 79)

Total number of ingredients: 9

## METHOD:

1. Combine all the ingredients except the zoodles, capers, and optional vegan cheese in a food processor or blender. Pulse for 1-2 minutes into a smooth pesto.
2. If desired, cook zoodles or zucchini slices for up to 4 minutes in a large skillet, with boiling water and a pinch of olive oil, over medium heat. Alternatively, the zoodles or zucchini slices can be used raw.
3. Melt the optional vegan cheese on a plate in the microwave for about 40 seconds, until it is melted and spreadable.
4. Serve the raw or cooked zoodles with the pesto, garnished with the chopped capers. Top the dish with the optional molten vegan cheese and add more salt and pepper to taste.
5. Serve and enjoy!
6. Alternatively, store the zoodle pesto salad in a multiple-compartment airtight container in the fridge and consume within 2 days. Store in the freezer for a maximum of 30 days and thaw at room temperature. Reheat without the zoodles in the microwave for up to 30 seconds.

# 10. Walnut & Mushroom Loaf

Serves: 10 | Prep Time: ~ 5 hours|

**Nutrition Information**
(per serving)
- Calories: 195 kcal
- Net Carbs: 2.9 g.
- Fat: 18.25 g.
- Protein: 4.5 g.
- Fiber: 2.1 g.
- Sugar: 1.7 g.

## INGREDIENTS:
- 2 tbsp. coconut oil
- 2 cups walnuts
- 3 portobello mushroom caps (stems removed)
- ½ cup green onion (sliced)
- 2 cups fresh baby spinach leaves

*Marinade:*
- 1 tbsp. balsamic vinegar
- 1 tbsp. soy sauce
- 1 tsp. cumin
- Pinch of Himalayan salt

Total number of ingredients: 9

## METHOD:

1. Grease a large cheese mold or loaf pan that fits in a dehydrator with coconut oil and set it aside.
2. In a medium-sized bowl, cover the walnuts with water and soak them for at least 8 hours. Rinse and drain the walnuts after soaking, and make sure no water is left.
3. Mix all the marinade ingredients in a small bowl until no lumps remain.
4. Cut the portobello mushroom caps into small pieces. Add to the marinade bowl and stir until all pieces are evenly coated. Set the mushrooms aside for 30 minutes.
5. After 30 minutes, put the walnuts into a food processor or blender and pulse into tiny bits. Add the marinated mushroom pieces and green onion and continue pulsing the ingredients into a smooth mixture with tiny chunks. This should take about 2 minutes.
6. Transfer the mixture into the cheese mold and sprinkle with some additional salt.
7. Cover the mold with parchment paper and place the walnut and mushroom loaf into a dehydrator. Dehydrate the loaf at 90°F/32°C for about 2 hours.
8. After 2 hours, flip the mold upside down and dehydrate for another 2 hours.
9. Take the loaf out of the mold and cut it into 10 slices or chunks.
10. Serve each slice with a handful of baby spinach leaves and enjoy!
11. Alternatively, store the walnut and mushroom loaf slices in an airtight container in the fridge and consume within 3 days.

# 11. Savory Coconut Pancake

**Nutrition Information**
(per serving)
- Calories: 281 kcal
- Net Carbs: 9.85 g.
- Fat: 22.05 g.
- Protein: 8.2 g.
- Fiber: 16 g.
- Sugar: 3.3 g.

## INGREDIENTS:
- ¼ cup coconut flour
- ¼ cup water
- ¼ cup green onion (diced)
- 1 tbsp. flax seeds (ground)
- ¼ tsp. baking powder
- ¼ tsp. turmeric
- Sea salt and black pepper to taste
- 1 tsp. coconut oil
- Handful fresh rocket

Total number of ingredients: 10

## METHOD:

1. In a medium-sized bowl, mix all the ingredients except the coconut oil and rocket together until no lumps remain. Set the bowl aside and allow the mixture to sit for up to 5 minutes.
2. Put a medium-sized skillet over medium-low heat and add the coconut oil.
3. When the oil is shimmering, pour in the coconut flour mixture and allow the pancake to firm up.
4. Flip the pancake carefully by loosening the edges with a spatula, then covering the skillet with a plate, turning the skillet upside down, and sliding the pancake back into the skillet.
5. Cook the pancake for another 2 minutes. If desired, add seasonings to taste.
6. Serve the coconut pancake warm, garnished with a handful of rocket, and enjoy!
7. Alternatively, store the pancake in an airtight container in the fridge and consume within 3 days. Store for a maximum of 60 days in the freezer and thaw at room temperature before serving.

*Tip: This pancake makes a great on-the-go lunch and goes well with spinach or a low-carb cheese!*

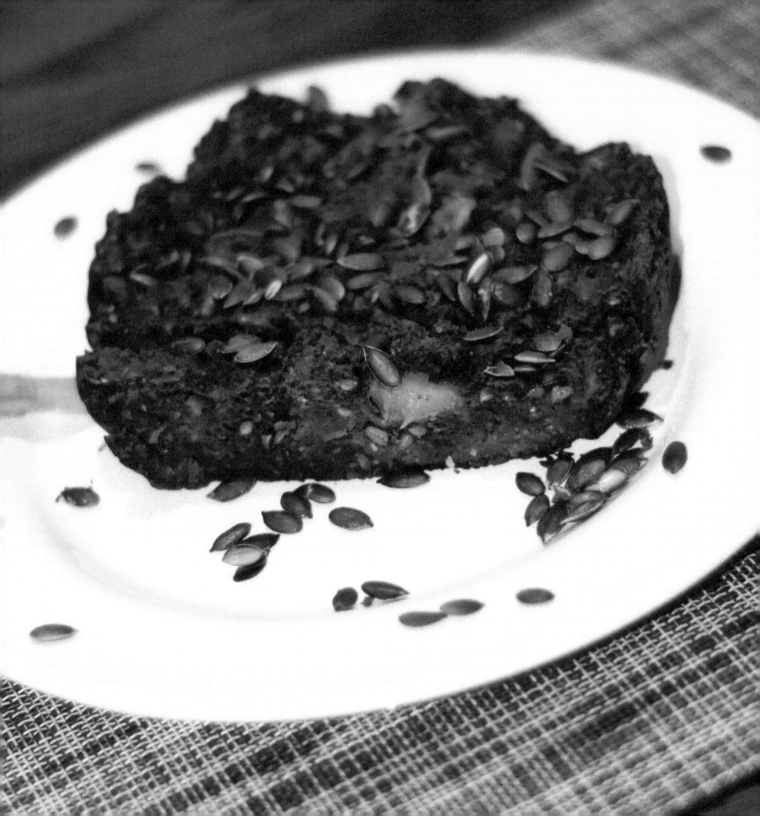

# 12. Flourless Bread

Serves: 12 | Prep Time: ~20 min |

**Nutrition Information**
(per serving)
- Calories: 191 kcal
- Net Carbs: 3.3 g.
- Fat: 14.7 g.
- Protein: 10.8 g.
- Fiber: 2.9 g.
- Sugar: 1 g.

## INGREDIENTS:
- 1 tsp. coconut oil
- 6 tbsp. water
- 2 tbsp. flax seed (ground)
- 1 cup almond butter
- 1 cup pumpkin (pitted, diced, cooked. Alternatively, use canned pumpkin puree.)
- 1 ½ tsp. baking powder
- ½ tsp. cinnamon
- 1 cup organic soy protein (vanilla flavor)
- ¼ cup pumpkin seeds (raw or roasted)
- Optional: ½ tsp. nutmeg

Total number of ingredients: 10

## METHOD:
1. Preheat the oven to 320°F/160°C.
2. Line a large loaf pan with parchment paper and grease the paper with the coconut oil.
3. In a small bowl, combine the water with the flax seeds. Allow the seeds to soak for about 10 minutes.
4. After 10 minutes, put all the ingredients except the roasted pumpkin seeds in a blender or food processor. If desired, include the optional nut-meg. Pulse until ingredients are combined into a smooth batter, scraping the sides of the blender or food processor if necessary.
5. Transfer the batter into the loaf pan and allow the mixture to sit for a few minutes.
6. Put the loaf pan in the oven and bake the bread for 20 minutes. Remove the bread and top it with the pumpkin seeds, then bake for another 15-20 minutes, or until a knife comes out clean. Take the loaf pan out of the oven and allow the bread to cool.
7. Transfer the bread to a cutting board and slice it into 12 slices.
8. Serve warm or cold and enjoy!
9. Alternatively, store the bread in an airtight container in the fridge and consume within 4 days. Store for a maximum of 60 days in the freezer and thaw at room temperature before serving.

*Tip: Serve the bread with a vegan cheese or guacamole!*

# 13. Tofu Stir-Fry Noodle Bowl ⑧

Serves: 2 | Prep Time: ~25 min |

**Nutrition Information**
(per serving)
- Calories: 558 kcal
- Net Carbs: 9.8 g.
- Fat: 46.65 g.
- Protein: 21.8 g.
- Fiber: 17.1 g.
- Sugar: 7.9 g.

## INGREDIENTS:
- 1 (12 oz. pack) extra firm tofu
  (drained, cubed)
- 2 (7 oz. packs) shirataki noodles
- 1 tbsp. coconut oil
- 1 tbsp. sesame oil
- 1 red bell pepper (seeded, chopped)
- 1 cup bok choi (finely chopped)

*Sauce:*
- 2 tbsp. low-sodium soy sauce
- ½ tbsp. rice vinegar
- 1 tsp. chili garlic paste (page 31)
- 1-inch piece ginger (finely chopped)
- 1 tsp. low-carb maple syrup
- 1 tsp. lemon juice
- 2 tsp. sesame oil

*Toppings:*
- ½ cup pickled red cabbage
- 1 medium Hass avocado
  (peeled, pitted, sliced)
- ¼ cup toasted sesame seeds

Total number of ingredients: 15

## METHOD:

1. In a medium-sized bowl, rinse the shirataki noodles with cold water, drain, and set aside.
2. Add the sauce ingredients to another medium-sized bowl and whisk thoroughly until smooth. Set the bowl aside.
3. Warm a large skillet over medium-high heat.
4. Add the coconut oil and sesame oil and stir until the bottom of the skillet is coated and the oil is shimmering.
5. Add the tofu cubes and the chopped bell pepper to the skillet. Stir fry until the tofu cubes start to brown.
6. Add the bok choi, noodles, and sauce to the skillet and stir fry for another 5 minutes.
7. Take the skillet off the heat and divide the tofu stir fry between two bowls.
8. Add some pickled red cabbage and avocado slices to each serving, garnish with sesame seeds, and enjoy!
9. Alternatively, store the tofu stir-fry noodle bowl without the toppings in an airtight container in the fridge. Consume within 3 days. Store in the freezer for a maximum of 30 days and thaw at room temperature. Use a microwave, toaster oven, or skillet to reheat the tofu stir-fry noodle bowl, then add fresh garnishes.

# 14. Spicy Satay Tofu Salad

**Serves: 2 | Prep Time: ~35 min |**

## Nutrition Information
(per serving)
- Calories: 656.1 kcal
- Net Carbs: 11.5 g.
- Fat: 54.4 g.
- Protein: 29 g.
- Fiber: 6.85 g.
- Sugar: 6 g.

## INGREDIENTS:
- 1 (12 oz. pack) extra firm tofu (drained and cubed)
- ¼ cup peanut butter (page 30)
- ½ tbsp. smoked paprika
- 1 tbsp. sesame oil
- ¼ tbsp. red chili flakes
- 2 drops liquid smoke
- 2 tbsp. water
- 1 tbsp. black sesame seeds

*Salad:*
- 4 cups fresh baby spinach leaves (rinsed, drained)
- ¼ cup fresh mint leaves (chopped)
- 2 tbsp. lemon juice
- 2 tbsp. avocado oil
- ¼ cup roasted cashews (unsalted)

Total number of ingredients: 13

## METHOD:

1. Preheat the oven to 400°F/200°C and line a baking tray with parchment paper.
2. Put the peanut butter, paprika, sesame oil, chili flakes and liquid smoke into a large bowl.
3. Add the water to the bowl and mix thoroughly until all the ingredients are combined.
4. Put the tofu cubes in the bowl with the peanut butter mixture and stir gently until all cubes are evenly covered.
5. Transfer the covered tofu cubes onto the baking tray, spread them out evenly, and sprinkle the sesame seeds over them.
6. Put the baking tray in the oven and bake the tofu cubes for 18 minutes, or until browned and firm.
7. Mix all the salad ingredients together in a large bowl.
8. Take the tofu out of the oven and let the cubes cool for about 2 minutes.
9. Divide the salad between two bowls, serve the tofu on top and enjoy!
10. Alternatively, store the peanut butter tofu and salad separately in airtight containers in the fridge and consume within 2 days. Store the tofu in the freezer for a maximum of 30 days and thaw at room temperature. Use a microwave, toaster oven, or frying pan to reheat the tofu. Do not reheat the salad.

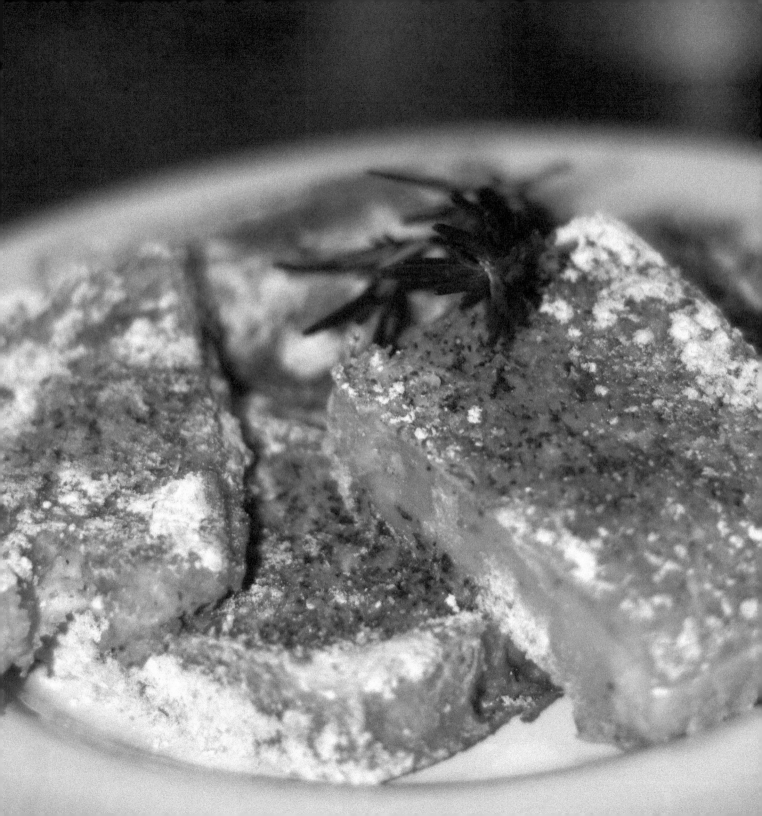

# 15. Lemon Rosemary Almond Slices

**Nutrition Information**
(per serving)
- Calories: 442 kcal
- Net Carbs: 5.2 g.
- Fat: 38.4 g.
- Protein: 17.9 g.
- Fiber: 6.2 g.
- Sugar: 3.2 g.

## INGREDIENTS:
- 1 (12 oz. pack) extra firm tofu (drained)
- 1 cup full-fat coconut milk
- 1 cup almond flour

*Crust:*
- ½ cup raw almonds
- 1 sprig rosemary leaves (stems removed)
- 1 tbsp. organic lemon zest
- 1 tsp. Himalayan salt
- 1 garlic clove (minced)
- 1 tsp. ground black pepper

Total number of ingredients: 9

## METHOD:

1. Preheat the oven to 400°F/200°C and line a baking tray with parchment paper.
2. Press the tofu down on a plate to get rid of any excess water and cut the block into 8 slices. Set the slices aside.
3. Put the almonds and rosemary into a food processor and process until chunky.
4. Add the remaining crust ingredients to the food processor and pulse until thoroughly combined.
5. Transfer mixture to a bowl. Pour the coconut milk into another medium-sized bowl and put the almond flour in a third medium-sized bowl.
6. Take a slice of tofu, dip each side in the bowl with almond flour and shake off any excess.
7. Dip the slice of flour-covered tofu into the coconut milk, and finally, dip it into the bowl with the lemon rosemary crust mix.
8. Place the coated slice of tofu onto the baking tray and repeat the process for all the tofu slices. Make sure to leave sufficient space between each slice.
9. Put the tray in the oven and bake the tofu slices for about 20 minutes, until browned and crispy.
10. Take the baking tray out of the oven and let the slices cool down for about a minute.
11. Serve with a light salad of greens as a side dish and enjoy!
12. Alternatively, store the tofu slices in an airtight container in the fridge and consume within 3 days. Store in the freezer for a maximum of 30 days and thaw at room temperature. Use a microwave, toaster oven, or frying pan to reheat the tofu slices.

# 16. California Scramble Bowl ⑧

Serves: 2 | Prep Time: ~20 min |

**Nutrition Information**
(per serving)
- Calories: 428 kcal
- Net Carbs: 9.3 g.
- Fat: 34.5 g.
- Protein: 18.2 g.
- Fiber: 11.3 g.
- Sugar: 5.2 g.

## INGREDIENTS:
- 1 (10 oz. pack) extra firm smoked tofu (drained, scrambled)
- 2 tbsp. olive oil
- ½ green onion (finely chopped)
- 2 cloves garlic (minced)
- 1 jalapeño (seeded, finely chopped)
- 1 tsp. dried oregano
- ½ tsp. ground cumin
- ½ tsp. smoked paprika

*Salad:*
- 4 cups iceberg lettuce (chopped)
- ¼ cup fresh cilantro (chopped)
- 1 large Hass avocado (peeled, pitted, sliced)
- 2 tbsp. lemon juice

Total number of ingredients: 12

## METHOD:

1. Put a large skillet over medium-high heat and add the olive oil.
2. Once oil is warm and shimmering, add the onion and garlic. Stir fry until the ingredients start to caramelize.
3. Stir in the tofu scramble, chopped jalapeño, oregano, cumin, and smoked paprika.
4. Stir-fry for about 7 minutes then turn off the heat.
5. Divide the lettuce between two medium-sized bowls. Add half of the tofu scramble, chopped cilantro and avocado slices to each.
6. Top the avocado slices with the lemon juice, serve and enjoy!
7. Alternatively, store the tofu scramble and salad separately in a two-compartment airtight container in the fridge and consume within 2 days. Store the California tofu scramble in the freezer for a maximum of 30 days and thaw at room temperature. Use a microwave, toaster oven, or skillet to reheat the tofu scramble. Do not reheat the salad.

# 17. Steamed Eggplant with Cashew Dressing

**Nutrition Information**
(per serving)
- Calories: 168.5 kcal
- Net Carbs: 9.8 g.
- Fat: 11.5 g.
- Protein: 4.9 g.
- Fiber: 8.88 g.
- Sugar: 9.9 g.

## INGREDIENTS:
- 3 small eggplants
- ¼ cup vegan mozzarella cheese (page 79)
- 1 tbsp. water
- 1 tbsp. soy sauce
- 1 tbsp. chili oil
- 1 tbsp. toasted sesame seeds
- ½ shallot (minced)
- 1 tbsp. dried cilantro

Total number of ingredients: 8

## METHOD:

1. Fill a large pot (with a steamer on top) halfway with water and put it over medium-high heat.
2. Halve the eggplants lengthwise and put them in the steamer basket once the water is simmering.
3. Steam the eggplant halves for about 15 minutes, until they are soft and tender.
4. Meanwhile, add the vegan mozzarella, water, soy sauce, and chili oil to a medium-sized bowl and whisk thoroughly until all ingredients are combined.
5. Once the eggplant halves are cooked, remove them from the heat and arrange them on a medium platter.
6. Drizzle the mozzarella mixture over the eggplant halves and top with the sesame seeds, minced shallot and cilantro. Serve warm and enjoy!
7. Alternatively, store the cooked eggplant in an airtight container in the fridge and consume within 2 days. Store in the freezer for a maximum of 30 days and thaw at room temperature. Use a toaster oven or frying pan to reheat the eggplant.

# 18. Eggplant Chips 'n Dips ⊚

Serves: 12 | Prep Time: ~45 min |

**Nutrition Information**
(per serving)
- Calories: 134 kcal
- Net Carbs: 6.45 g.
- Fat: 10.1 g.
- Protein: 3.3 g.
- Fiber: 5.6 g.
- Sugar: 5.4 g.

## INGREDIENTS:
- 2 large eggplants
- 1 tsp. salt
- 2 tbsp. olive oil
- 1 garlic clove (minced)
- 1 tbsp. oregano
- 1 tbsp. smoked paprika
- 1 tsp. ground cumin

*Salad:*
- 4 cups fresh baby spinach
  (rinsed and drained)
- ½ cup pickled red cabbage (chopped)
- ½ red onion (finely chopped)
- 1 tbsp. lemon juice

*Dips:*
- ½ cup mozzarella cheese (page 79)
- ½ cup guacamole (page 32)
- ½ cup Mexican salsa (page 33)

Total number of ingredients: 14

## METHOD:

1. Preheat the oven to 350°F/175°C.
2. Cut the eggplants lengthwise into ¼ inch slices and lay them out in one layer on a baking tray lined with parchment paper.
3. Sprinkle the salt on the layer of eggplant slices and set them aside for about an hour to let the salt dry out the slices. Gently remove excess moisture with paper towels.
4. In a medium-sized bowl, put the olive oil, minced garlic, oregano, smoked paprika, and cumin. Mix thoroughly until everything is combined.
5. Brush both sides of the eggplant slices with the spice mixture, making sure all slices are evenly coated.
6. Spread out the eggplant slices in one layer back onto the baking tray, leaving space between each slice.
7. Put the baking tray in the oven and bake for about 25 to 30 minutes, until browned and crispy.
8. Toss all salad ingredients in a large bowl, then divide between two medium-sized bowls.
9. Take the baking tray from the oven and let the chips cool for a minute.
10. Put half of the eggplant chips into each bowl and serve with half of each dip. Enjoy!
11. Alternatively, store the eggplant chips, toppings, and salad separately in airtight containers or a multiple compartment container in the fridge. Consume within 2 days. Store the eggplant chips in the freezer for a maximum of 30 days and thaw at room temperature. Reheat eggplant chips in a toaster oven for a few minutes, and serve with fresh salad and dips.

# 1. Feta Cheese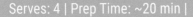

Serves: 4 | Prep Time: ~20 min |

**Nutrition Information**
(per serving)
- Calories: 101 kcal
- Net Carbs: 3.8 g.
- Fat: 4.9 g.
- Protein: 10.3 g.
- Fiber:1.4 g.
- Sugar: 0.7 g.

## INGREDIENTS:
- 1 13-oz. block extra firm tofu (drained)
- 3 cups water
- ¼ cup apple cider vinegar
- 2 tbsp. dark miso paste
- 1 tsp. ground black pepper
- 2 garlic cloves
- 1 tbsp. sun dried tomatoes (chopped)
- 2 tsp. Himalayan salt

Total number of ingredients: 8

## METHOD:

1. Cut the tofu into ½-inch cubes and put them into a medium-sized saucepan with 2 cups of water.
2. Bring the water to a boil over medium-high heat, take the saucepan off the heat immediately, drain half of the water, and set aside to let it cool down.
3. Pour the vinegar, miso paste, pepper, salt, and the remaining 1 cup of water into a blender or food processor. Blend until everything is well combined.
4. Pour the liquid from the blender into an airtight container. Add the garlic cloves, sundried tomatoes, and the tofu (including the water) to the container.
5. Give the feta cheese a good stir and then store in the fridge or freezer for at least 4 hours before serving.
6. Serve with low-carb crackers, or, enjoy this delicious feta cheese in a healthy salad!
7. Alternatively, store the cheese in an airtight container in the fridge and consume within 6 days. Store for a maximum of 30 days in the freezer and thaw at room temperature.

## CHEESES

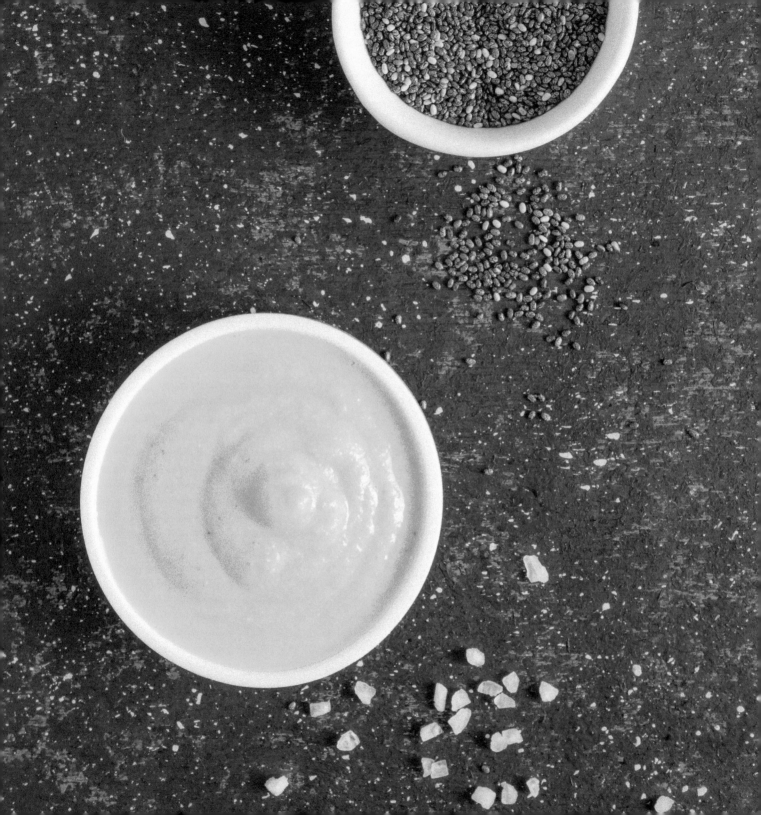

# 2. Smokey Cheddar Cheese ⊚

**Nutrition Information**
(per serving)
- Calories: 249 kcal
- Net Carbs: 6.9 g.
- Fat: 21.7 g.
- Protein: 6.1 g.
- Fiber: 4.3 g.
- Sugar: 2.6 g.

## INGREDIENTS:
- 1 cup raw cashews (unsalted)
- 1 cup macadamia nuts (unsalted)
- 4 tsp. tapioca starch
- 1 cup water
- ¼ cup fresh lime juice
- ¼ cup tahini
- ½ tsp. liquid smoke
- ¼ cup paprika powder
- ½ tsp. ground mustard seeds
- 2 tbsp. onion powder
- 1 tsp. Himalayan salt
- ½ tsp. chili powder
- 1 tbsp. coconut oil

Total number of ingredients: 13

## METHOD:

1. Cover the cashews with water in a small bowl and let sit for 4 to 6 hours. Rinse and drain the cashews after soaking. Make sure no water is left.
2. Mix the tapioca starch with the cup of water in a small saucepan. Heat the pan over medium heat.
3. Bring the water with tapioca starch to a boil. After 1 minute, take the saucepan off the heat and set the mixture aside to cool down.
4. Put all the remaining ingredients—except the coconut oil—in a blender or food processor. Blend until these ingredients are combined into a smooth mixture.
5. Stir in the tapioca starch with water and blend again until all ingredients have fully incorporated.
6. Grease a medium-sized bowl with the coconut oil to prevent the cheese from sticking to the edges. Gently pour the mixture into the bowl.
7. Refrigerate the bowl, uncovered, for about 3 hours until the cheese is firm and ready to enjoy!
8. Alternatively, store the cheese in an airtight container in the fridge and consume within 6 days. Store for a maximum of 60 days in the freezer and thaw at room temperature.

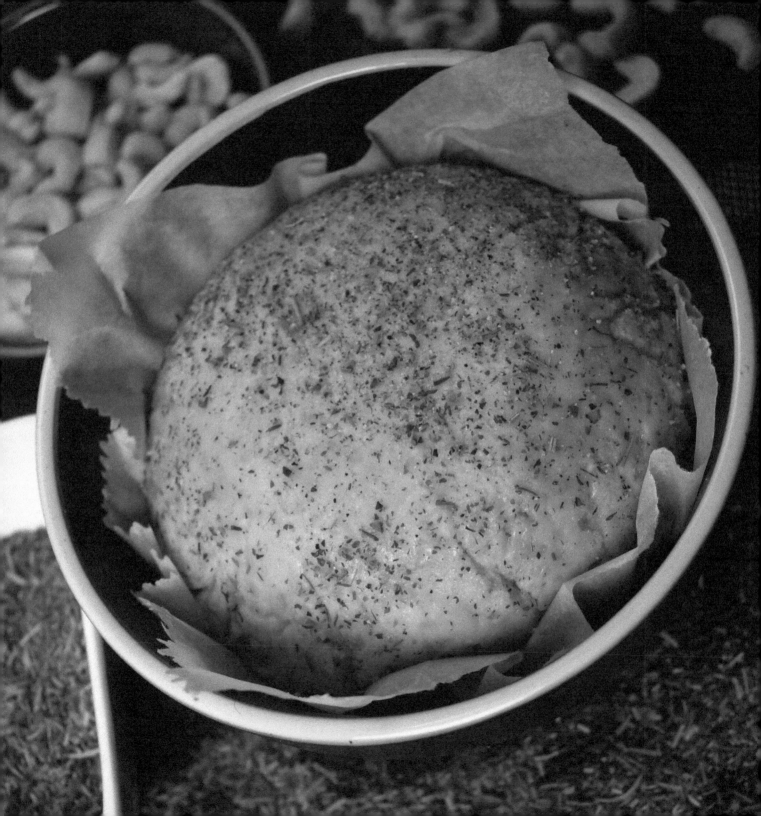

# 3. Mozzarella Cheese ⊛

**Serves: 16 / 1 block of cheese | Prep Time: ~20 min |**

**Nutrition Information**
(per serving)
- Calories: 101 kcal
- Net Carbs: 2.1 g.
- Fat: 9.2 g.
- Protein: 2.2 g.
- Fiber: 0.9 g.
- Sugar: 0.9 g.

## INGREDIENTS:
- 1 cup raw cashews (unsalted)
- ½ cup macadamia nuts (unsalted)
- ½ cup pine nuts
- ½ cup water
- ½ tbsp. coconut oil
- 2 tbsp. agar-agar
- 1 tsp. fresh lime juice
- 1 tsp. Himalayan salt
- Optional: ½ tsp. light miso paste

Total number of ingredients: 9

## METHOD:

1. Cover the cashews with water in a small bowl and let sit for 4 to 6 hours. Rinse and drain the cashews after soaking. Make sure no water is left.
2. Mix the agar-agar with the ½ cup of water in a small saucepan. Put the pan over medium heat.
3. Bring the agar-agar mixture to a boil. After 1 minute, take it off the heat and set the mixture aside to cool down.
4. Put all the other ingredients—except the coconut oil—in a blender or food processor. Blend until everything is well combined.
5. Add the agar-agar with water and blend again until all ingredients have been fully incorporated.
6. Grease a medium-sized bowl with the coconut oil to prevent the cheese from sticking to the edges. Gently transfer the cheese mixture into the bowl by using a spatula.
7. Refrigerate the bowl, uncovered, for about 3 hours until the cheese is firm; then serve and enjoy!
8. Alternatively, store the cheese in an airtight container in the fridge. Consume within 6 days. Store for a maximum of 60 days in the freezer and thaw at room temperature.

# 4. Nut Free Nacho Dip

**Nutrition Information**
(per serving)
- Calories: 135 kcal
- Net Carbs: 3.5 g.
- Fat: 12.3 g.
- Protein: 1.8 g.
- Fiber: 5.4 g.
- Sugar: 2.7 g.

## INGREDIENTS:
- 1 large eggplant (peeled and cubed)
- 2 medium Hass avocados
  (peeled, pitted, and halved)
- ¼ cup MCT oil
- 2 tsp. nutritional yeast
- 1 jalapeno pepper
- 1 red onion (diced)
- 1 garlic clove (halved)
- ¼ cup fresh cilantro (chopped)
- 1 tbsp. paprika powder
- 1 tsp. cumin seeds
- 1 tsp. dried oregano
- ½ tsp. Himalayan salt

Total number of ingredients: 12

## METHOD:
1. Slice the jalapeno in half lengthwise; remove the seeds, stem, and placenta, and discard.
2. Put the jalapeno and all other ingredients in a food processor or blender.
3. Mix everything into a smooth mixture. Use a spatula to scrape down the sides of the blender to make sure everything gets mixed evenly.
4. Transfer the dip to an airtight container.
5. Serve, share, and enjoy!
6. Alternatively, store the cheese in an airtight container in the fridge and consume within 2 days.

*Tip: Serve with some celery sticks!*

# 5. Black Olive & Thyme Cheese Spread

**Nutrition Information**
(per serving)
- Calories: 118 kcal
- Net Carbs: 0.7 g.
- Fat: 11.9 g.
- Protein: 2 g.
- Fiber: 1.4 g.
- Sugar: 0.7 g.

## INGREDIENTS:
- 1 cup macadamia nuts (unsalted)
- 1 cup pine nuts
- 1 tsp. thyme (finely chopped)
- 1 tsp. rosemary (finely chopped)
- 2 tsp. nutritional yeast
- 1 tsp. Himalayan salt
- 10 black olives (pitted, finely chopped)

Total number of ingredients: 7

## METHOD:

1. Preheat the oven to 350°F/175°C, and line a baking sheet with parchment paper.
2. Put the nuts on a baking sheet, and spread them out so they can roast evenly. Transfer the baking sheet to the oven and roast the nuts for about 8 minutes, until slightly browned.
3. Take the nuts out of the oven and set aside for about 4 minutes, allowing them to cool down.
4. Add all ingredients to a blender and process until everything combines into a smooth mixture. Use a spatula to scrape down the sides of the blender container in between blending to make sure everything gets mixed evenly.
5. Serve, share, and enjoy!
6. Alternatively, store the cheese in an airtight container in the fridge and consume within 6 days. Store for a maximum of 60 days in the freezer and thaw at room temperature.

*Tip: Serve with some low-carb crackers!*

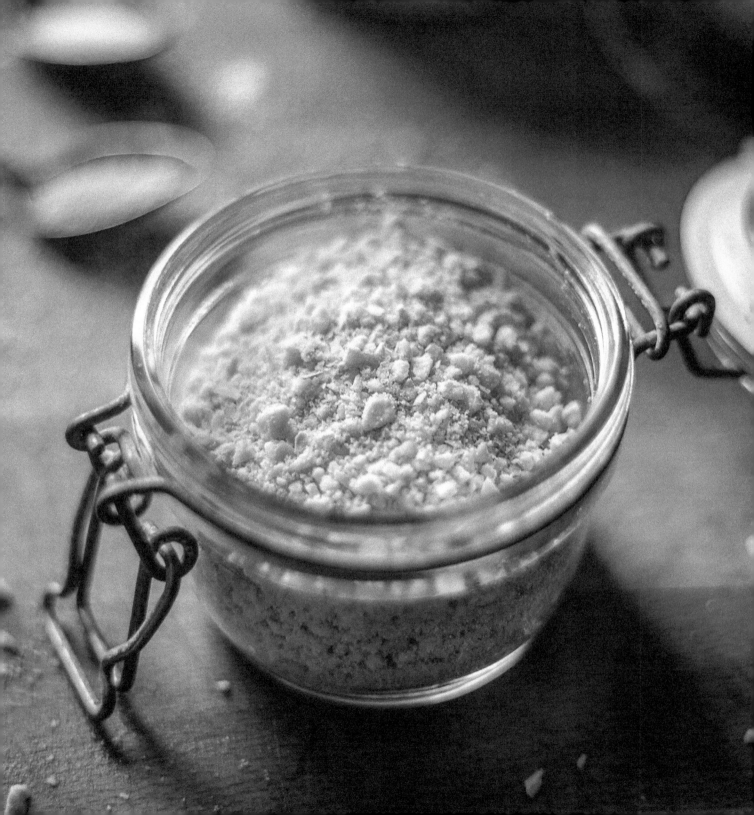

# 6. Truffle Parmesan Cheese ⊚

Serves: 8 | Prep Time: ~30 min |

**Nutrition Information**
(per serving)
- Calories: 202 kcal
- Net Carbs: 4.4 g.
- Fat: 18.7 g.
- Protein: 4 g.
- Fiber: 1.8 g.
- Sugar: 1.8 g.

## INGREDIENTS:
- 1 cup macadamia nuts (unsalted)
- 1 cup raw cashews (unsalted)
- 2 garlic cloves
- ½ tbsp. nutritional yeast
- 2 tbsp. truffle oil
- 1 tsp. agar-agar
- 1 tsp. fresh lime juice
- Optional: 1 tsp. dark miso paste

Total number of ingredients: 8

## METHOD:

1. Cover the cashews with water in a small bowl and let sit for 4 to 6 hours. Rinse and drain the cashews after soaking. Make sure no water is left.
2. Preheat the oven to 350°F/175°C, and line a baking sheet with parchment paper.
3. Put the macadamia nuts on a baking sheet and spread them out, so they can roast evenly.
4. Transfer the baking sheet to the oven and roast the macadamia nuts for about 8 minutes, until slightly browned.
5. Take the nuts out of the oven and set them aside, allowing them to cool down.
6. Grease a medium shallow baking dish with ½ tablespoon of truffle oil.
7. Add the soaked cashews, roasted macadamia nuts, and all the remaining ingredients to a blender or food processor. Blend everything into a crumbly mixture.
8. Transfer the crumbly parmesan into the baking dish, spread it out evenly, and firmly press it down until it has fused together into an even layer of cheese.
9. Cover the baking dish with aluminum foil and refrigerate the cheese for 8 hours or until the parmesan is firm.
10. Serve or store the cheese in an airtight container in the fridge and consume within 6 days. Store for a maximum of 60 days in the freezer and thaw at room temperature.

# 7. Gorgonzola 'Blue' Cheese

Serves: 16 | Prep Time: ~24 hours |

**Nutrition Information**
(per serving)
- Calories: 101 kcal
- Net Carbs: 2 g.
- Fat: 9.3 g.
- Protein: 2.3 g.
- Fiber: 1 g.
- Sugar: 0.9 g.

## INGREDIENTS:
- ½ cup macadamia nuts (unsalted)
- ½ cup pine nuts
- 1 cup raw cashews (unsalted)
- 1 capsule acidophilus
  (probiotic cheese culture)
- ½ tbsp. MCT oil
- ¼ cup unsweetened almond milk
- 1 tsp. ground black pepper
- 1 tsp. Himalayan salt
- 1 tsp. spirulina powder

Total number of ingredients: 9

## METHOD:

1. Cover the cashews with water in a small bowl and let sit for 4 to 6 hours. Rinse and drain the cashews after soaking. Make sure no water is left.
2. Preheat the oven to 350°F/175°C, and line a baking sheet with parchment paper.
3. Spread the macadamia and pine nuts out on the baking sheet so they can roast evenly.
4. Put the baking sheet into the oven and roast the nuts for 8 minutes, until they are slightly browned.
5. Take the nuts out of the oven and allow them to cool down.
6. Grease a 3-inch cheese mold with the MCT oil and set it aside.
7. Add all ingredients—except the spirulina—to the blender or food processor. Blend on medium speed into a smooth mixture. Use a spatula to scrape down the sides of the blender to make sure all the ingredients get incorporated.
8. Transfer the cheese mixture into the greased cheese mold and sprinkle it with the spirulina powder. Use a small teaspoon to create blue marble veins on the cheese, and then cover the mold with parchment paper.
9. Place the cheese into a dehydrator and dehydrate the cheese at 90°F/32°C for 24 hours.
10. Transfer the dehydrated cheese in the covered mold to the fridge. Allow the cheese to refrigerate for 12 hours.
11. Remove the cheese from the mold to serve in this condition, or, age the cheese in a wine cooler for up to 3 weeks. In case of aging the cheese, rub the outsides of the cheese with fresh sea salt. Refresh the salt every 2 days to prevent any mold. The cheese will develop a blue cheese-like taste, and by aging it, the cheese becomes even more delicious.
12. If the cheese is not aged, store it in airtight container and consume within 6 days.
13. Store the aged cheese in an airtight container and consume within 6 days, or for a maximum of 60 days in the freezer and thaw at room temperature.

# 8. Smoked Chipotle Cream Cheese

**Nutrition Information**
(per serving)
- Calories: 223 kcal
- Net Carbs: 2.9 g.
- Fat: 21.4 g.
- Protein: 4.3 g.
- Fiber: 3.5 g.
- Sugar: 1.9 g.

## INGREDIENTS:
- 1 cup macadamia nuts (unsalted)
- ½ cup walnuts
- ½ cup pine nuts
- ¼ cup fresh lemon juice
- 1 tbsp. smoked chipotle pepper
- 1 garlic clove
- 2 tbsp. paprika powder
- ½ tbsp. dried cilantro
- ½ tbsp. dried oregano
- ½ tbsp. dried thyme
- ½ tbsp. dried sweet basil
- 1 tsp. ground cumin

Total number of ingredients: 12

## METHOD:

1. Add all ingredients to a blender or food processor. Blend everything into a smooth mixture. Use a spatula to scrape down the sides of the blender to make sure all the ingredients get incorporated.
2. Serve right away and enjoy!
3. Alternatively, store the cheese in an airtight container in the fridge and consume within 6 days. Store for a maximum of 60 days in the freezer and thaw at room temperature.

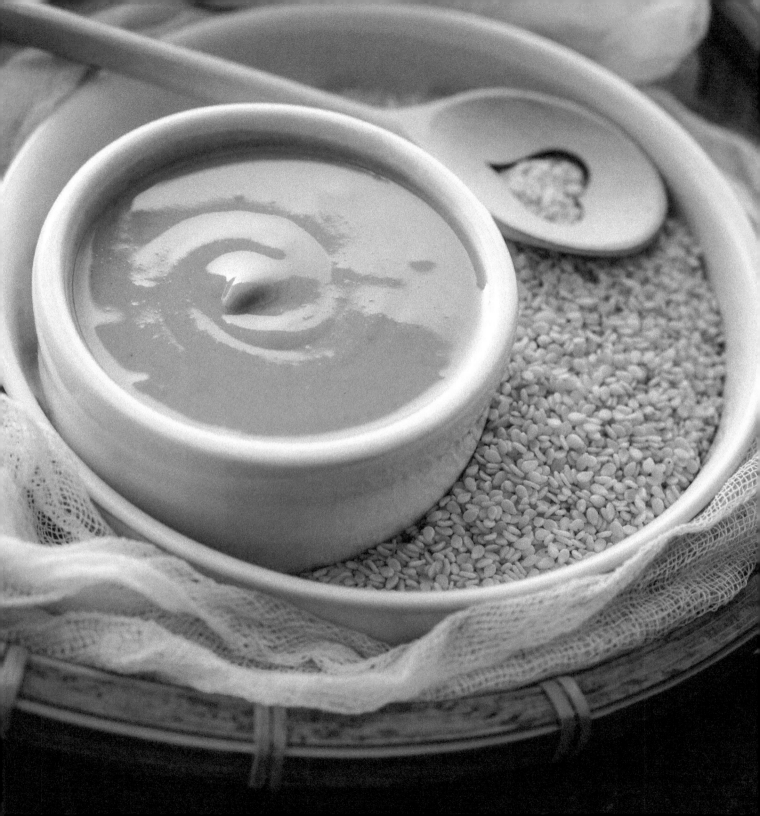

# 9. Sesame Cheese Spread

Serves: 8 | Prep Time: ~20 min |

**Nutrition Information**
(per serving)
- Calories: 111 kcal
- Net Carbs: 3.4 g.
- Fat: 9 g.
- Protein: 3.7 g.
- Fiber: 2.7 g.
- Sugar: 1 g.

## INGREDIENTS:
- 1 cup sesame seeds
- 3 tbsp. lemon juice
- 1 tsp. Himalayan salt
- ½ tsp. rice syrup
- 1 tsp. ground black pepper
- ¼ cup fresh lovage (chopped)
- ¼ cup fresh mint (chopped)

Total number of ingredients: 7

## METHOD:

1. Cover the sesame seeds in a small bowl filled with water and add 1 tablespoon of lemon juice. Soak the sesame seeds for 12 hours. Rinse and drain the seeds after soaking. Make sure no water is left.

2. Add all the ingredients to a blender or food processor. Blend everything into a smooth mixture. Use a spatula to scrape down the sides of the blender to make sure all the ingredients get incorporated.

3. Serve right away, as a dip for veggies or with some low carb bread, and enjoy!

4. Alternatively, store the cheese in an airtight container in the fridge and consume within 4 days. Store for a maximum of 30 days in the freezer and thaw at room temperature.

# 10. Classic Cheese Sauce

**Nutrition Information**
(per serving)
- Calories: 183 kcal
- Net Carbs: 2.3 g.
- Fat: 16.8 g.
- Protein: 5.2 g.
- Fiber: 3.4 g.
- Sugar: 2.2 g.

## INGREDIENTS:
- 1 cup almonds
- 1 cup macadamia nuts (unsalted)
- 1 tbsp. white wine vinegar
- ½ cup sunflower seed butter
- 2 cups water
- ¼ cup fresh parsley (chopped)
- ¼ cup fresh lovage (chopped)
- 1 tsp. Himalayan salt
- 1 tbsp. nutritional yeast
- 1 tbsp. white truffle oil

Total number of ingredients: 10

## METHOD:

1. Cover the almonds and macadamia nuts with water in 2 separate small bowls. Soak the almonds for 12 hours, and the macadamia nuts for 4 to 6 hours. Rinse and drain the nuts after soaking. Make sure no water is left.

2. Transfer the 2 cups of water to a medium-sized saucepan and put it over medium heat. Bring the water to a boil and then add it to a blender or food processor.

3. Add the soaked nuts and the other remaining ingredients to the blender. Blend until everything is combined into a smooth mixture. Use a spatula to scrape down the sides of the blender to make sure all ingredients get incorporated.

4. Serve right away and enjoy!

5. Alternatively, store the cheese in an airtight container in the fridge and consume within 4 days. Store for a maximum of 30 days in the freezer and thaw at room temperature.

Tip: Serve with some low-carb crackers or celery sticks!

# 1. Special Zucchini Lasagna

Serves: 8 | Prep Time: ~45 min |

**Nutrition Information**
(per serving)
- Calories: 202 kcal
- Net Carbs: 5.4 g.
- Fat: 15.2 g.
- Protein: 10.1 g.
- Fiber: 3.4 g.
- Sugar: 2.8 g.

## INGREDIENTS:

*Walnut Sauce:*
- 1 cup walnuts (ground)
- 1 cup simple marinara sauce (page 28)
- ¼ cup sundried tomatoes (chopped)
- Optional: pinch of salt

*Tofu Ricotta:*
- 1 14-oz. package firm tofu (drained)
- ¼ cup fresh basil
- 1 tbsp. lemon juice
- 4 tbsp. nutritional yeast
- 2 small garlic cloves (minced)
- 1½ tbsp. olive oil
- Salt and pepper to taste

*Lasagna:*
- 2 zucchinis (thinly sliced)
- 2 cups simple marinara sauce (page 28)
- Salt and pepper to taste

Total number of ingredients: 16

## METHOD:

1. Preheat the oven to 375°F/190°C.
2. Add the walnut sauce ingredients to a blender. Blend the ingredients into an almost completely smooth mixture.
3. Transfer the mixture to a medium-sized bowl and set it aside.
4. Clean the blender container and then add all tofu ricotta ingredients. Blend until smooth.
5. Take a large loaf pan and add 2 cups of simple marinara sauce. Cover the sauce with the zucchini slices and top these with ⅓ of the tofu ricotta. Pour half of the walnut sauce on top.
6. Make another layer, starting with zucchini slices, then tofu ricotta, and then the remaining walnut sauce.
7. Finish the lasagna with a layer of zucchini slices and tofu ricotta. Top the dish with some additional salt and pepper to taste.
8. Transfer the lasagna to the oven and bake for 30-35 minutes.
9. Allow the lasagna to cool down before serving and enjoy!
10. Alternatively, store the lasagna in the fridge, using an airtight container, and consume within 4 days. Store in the freezer for a maximum of 30 days and thaw at room temperature. Use a microwave, toaster oven, or frying pan to reheat the lasagna.

*Tip: Incorporate vegan cheese in this lasagna. The final layer can also be topped with crushed walnuts.*

## DINNERS

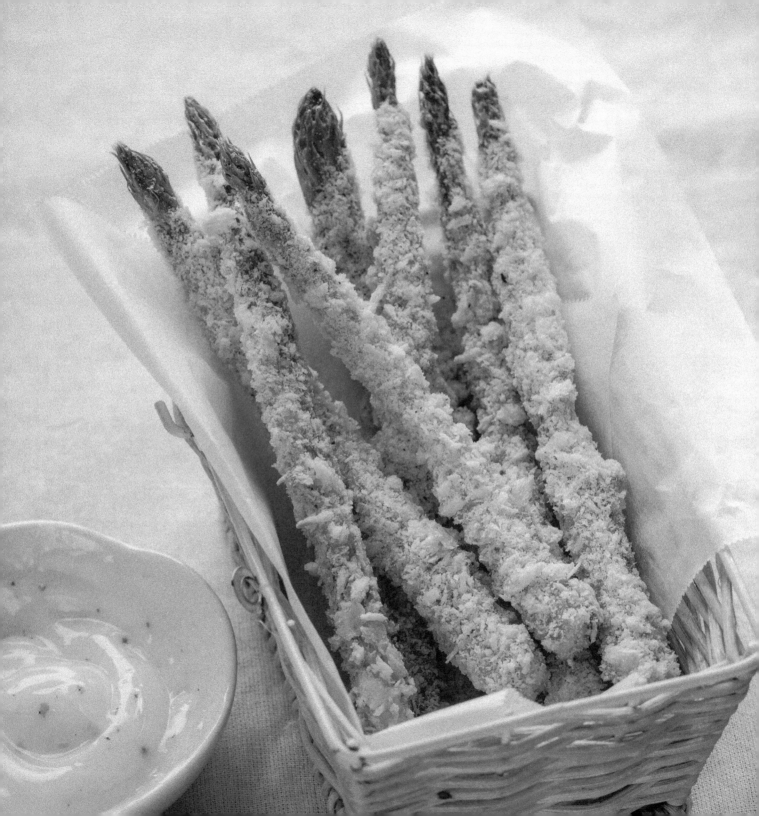

# 2. Crunchy Fried Asparagus

**Nutrition Information**
(per serving)
- Calories: 247 kcal
- Net Carbs: 3.8 g.
- Fat: 22 g.
- Protein: 7.7 g.
- Fiber: 4.2 g.
- Sugar: 1.6 g.

## INGREDIENTS:
- 10 asparagus spears
- 1 cup almond flour
- 2 tbsp. olive oil (alternatively use coconut oil)
- 1 tsp. sea salt
- ½ tsp. black pepper
- 1 tsp. smoked paprika
- 2 tsp. low-carb maple syrup
- 1½ tbsp. nutritional yeast

Total number of ingredients: 8

## METHOD:

1. Preheat the oven to 400°F/200°C, and line a baking sheet with parchment paper.
2. Cut the asparagus in half and transfer these halves to a medium-sized bowl.
3. Add the spices to the bowl and stir.
4. Take another medium-sized bowl or deep plate and add the flour and nutritional yeast. Stir and dip each asparagus fry in the dry mixture until coated.
5. Repeat this for all the fries. Then transfer the asparagus fries to the baking sheet.
6. Bake for 20-25 minutes, or until golden brown.
7. Serve the fries with a vegan dip sauce, and enjoy!
8. Alternatively, store the asparagus in the fridge, using an airtight container, and consume within 4 days. Store in the freezer for a maximum of 30 days and thaw at room temperature. Use a toaster oven or frying pan to reheat the fried asparagus.

*Tip: Add chili flakes, garlic powder, or white pepper for another taste.*

# 3. Green Curry Tofu with Cauliflower Rice

Serves: 4 | Prep Time: ~30 min |

**Nutrition Information**
(per serving)
- Calories: 177 kcal
- Net Carbs: 7.9 g.
- Fat: 13.5 g.
- Protein: 6 g.
- Fiber: 3.6 g.
- Sugar: 2.8 g.

## INGREDIENTS:
- 4 oz. silken tofu (drained)
- 1 tbsp. extra virgin coconut oil
- ½ cup coconut cream
- 1½ cups cauliflower rice (or blend 3-4 cups stemless cauliflower florets)
- 1 stalk lemongrass (sliced)
- ½ cup green peas
- ½ cup fresh basil
- ½ cup fresh cilantro
- 4 tbsp. soy sauce
- 3 garlic cloves (minced)
- 4 small green chilis
- 1½ tbsp. ginger
- 2 tbsp. green curry paste
- 1 lime
- 1 tbsp. canola oil
- ½ tsp. ground cumin
- ½ tsp. turmeric
- 1 tsp. salt

Total number of ingredients: 18

## METHOD:

1. Preheat the oven to 350°F/180°C, and line a baking sheet with parchment paper.
2. Cut the tofu into tiny cubes. Add the coconut oil and 1 tablespoon of soy sauce and make sure that all the cubes are greased.
3. Spread out the tofu on the baking sheet and transfer it to the oven. Bake the tofu cubes for 12-15 minutes.
4. Put all the ingredients—except the canola oil, cauliflower rice, remaining soy sauce, green peas, and salt—in a blender. Blend these ingredients into a liquid while adding 2 tablespoons of soy sauce.
5. Take a large skillet and heat it over medium heat. Add the canola oil, green curry paste, green peas, and the blended vegetables.
6. Stir in the coconut cream and let the mixture cook for about 5 minutes while stirring.
7. Add the cauliflower rice and the last tablespoon of soy sauce to the skillet.
8. Cook the mixture for 5 minutes while occasionally stirring.
9. Take the tofu out of the oven and sprinkle it with the salt.
10. Carefully add the tofu cubes to the dish and take the skillet off the heat.
11. Allow the food to cool down for about 10 minutes before serving and enjoy!
12. Alternatively, store the green curry tofu and the cauliflower rice, separated, in the fridge; use airtight containers and consume within 3 days. Store in the freezer for a maximum of 30 days and thaw at room temperature. Use a microwave or toaster oven to reheat green curry tofu with cauliflower rice.

*Note: Use less soy sauce and little or no salt for less sodium.*

*Tip: Add more low-carb (green) vegetables. Broccoli, green bell peppers, onions and green beans are great examples.*

# 4. Tofu Stir-Fry with Almond Bread

Serves: 4 | Prep Time: ~30 min |

**Nutrition Information**
(per serving)
- Calories: 380 kcal
- Net Carbs: 6.2 g.
- Fat: 30.6 g.
- Protein: 17.7 g.
- Fiber: 14.2 g.
- Sugar: 3.3 g.

## INGREDIENTS:

*Almond Bread:*
- 1 cup almond flour
- 4 tbsp. psyllium husk
- 2 flax eggs (page 27)
- 1½ tsp. baking powder
- 1½ cups hot water
- 1½ tbsp. apple cider vinegar
- Pinch of salt

*Tofu Scramble:*
- 1 tbsp. coconut oil
- 1 shallot (finely minced)
- 2 tsp. turmeric powder
- 1 tbsp. sweet paprika powder
- 2 tbsp. nutritional yeast
- Black pepper to taste
- Sea salt to taste
- 2 cups of kale (chopped)
- ½ cup of cherry tomatoes (halved)
- 1 8-oz. pack extra firm tofu

*Topping:*
- 1 medium Hass avocado (peeled, pitted, and sliced)
- Optional: 2 tbsp. roasted sesame seeds
- Optional: ½ cup spring onions (chopped)

Total number of ingredients: 20

## METHOD:

1. Preheat the oven to 400°F/200°C, and line a baking tray with parchment paper.
2. Mix all the dry bread ingredients in a medium-sized bowl.
3. Use a whisk and your hands to incorporate the flax eggs, water, and apple cider vinegar with the dry ingredients. A firm dough should be formed. Add more water if necessary.
4. Divide the dough into 4 flattened buns.
5. Transfer the buns to the baking tray and put this in the oven.
6. Bake the flat almond bread for about 40 minutes. Flip the buns after 20 minutes.
7. Take the baking tray out of the oven and allow the buns to cool off.
8. Chop the tofu into tiny cubes and set it aside.
9. Take a medium-sized skillet, put it over medium heat, and add the coconut oil.
10. Stir in the minced shallot, turmeric powder, paprika powder, yeast, pepper, and salt to taste.
11. Add the chopped kale and heat the ingredients for about 2 minutes while stirring.
12. Stir in the chopped tofu cubes and top the ingredients in the skillet with the halved cherry tomatoes. Stir the tofu scramble for a minute before turning off the heat.
13. Take the almond buns and top them with the tofu scramble.
14. Add the avocado slices and, if desired, garnish with the optional spring onions.
15. Sprinkle the optional sesame seeds over the toppings, serve, and enjoy!
16. Alternatively, store the bread and tofu scramble, separated, in the fridge. Use airtight containers and consume within 4 days. Store in the freezer for a maximum of 30 days and thaw at room temperature. Use a microwave, toaster oven, or frying pan to reheat the scramble.

*Tip: Top the almond bread with some pumpkin seeds or incorporate these into the dough.*

# 5. Creamy Mushroom soup with truffle oil

**Nutrition Information**
(per serving)
- Calories: 380 kcal
- Net Carbs: 11.6 g.
- Fat: 31.5 g.
- Protein: 11.5 g.
- Fiber: 6.1 g.
- Sugar: 3.9 g.

## INGREDIENTS:
- 2 cups white mushrooms (sliced)
- 1 cup portobello mushrooms
  (stems removed, chopped)
- 2 tbsp. olive oil
- 4 cups vegetable broth (page 29)
- 1 garlic clove (minced)
- ¼ cup almond butter
- ½ cup cashew butter
- 2 tsp. white truffle oil
- 2 shallots (minced)
- 1 celery rib (chopped)
- Handful of fresh thyme or parsley (chopped)
- Salt and black pepper to taste

Total number of ingredients: 13

## METHOD:

1. Take a medium-sized pot and put it over medium heat.
2. Add the olive oil, portobello mushrooms, 1 cup of the white mushrooms, garlic, shallots, and the celery to the pot.
3. Cook the ingredients for about 3 minutes, while continuously stirring with a wooden spoon.
4. Next add 2 cups of the vegetable broth and salt and pepper to taste.
5. In a blender container, add the almond butter, cashew butter, the remaining cup of white mushrooms and remaining 2 cups of vegetable broth.
6. Blend until smooth and creamy, and then add the mixture to the pot while stirring continuously to make sure it incorporates completely.
7. Add the truffle oil to the pot, stir thoroughly, cover, and allow the mixture to simmer for up to 15 minutes.
8. Turn off the heat, top the soup with the thyme (or parsley), give the soup a quick stir before serving, and enjoy!
9. Alternatively, store the soup in the fridge using an airtight container and consume within 3 days. Reheat the soup in the microwave for 1 minute.

*Tip: Incorporate sour cream or (vegan) half & half cream for an enhanced flavor!*

# 6. Zoodle chow ming with tofu scramble

**Nutrition Information**
(per serving)
- Calories: 169 kcal
- Net Carbs: 9.1 g.
- Fat: 9.7 g.
- Protein: 10.8 g.
- Fiber: 3.3 g.
- Sugar: 6.3 g.

## INGREDIENTS:
- 1 8-oz. block firm tofu (drained, cubed)
- 1½ tbsp sesame oil
- 1 medium zucchini
  (spiralized into zoodles)
- 2 cups Chinese cabbage (chopped)
- 1 cup bean sprouts
- 3 shallots or 3 green onions (diced)
- 2 garlic cloves (minced)
- ¼ cup water
- Optional: 1 medium carrot
  (matchsticks or julienned)

*Chow Ming Sauce:*
- 3 tbsp. soy sauce
- 1½ tbsp. Chinese cooking wine
- ¼ tsp. agar agar
- ½ tsp. sesame oil
- ½ tsp. stevia powder
- White pepper to taste

Total number of ingredients: 15

## METHOD:

1. In a small bowl, mix the sauce ingredients together with a teaspoon until no lumps remain.
2. Use a tablespoon of the chow ming sauce to marinate the tofu cubes and set the rest of the sauce aside.
3. Toss the tofu cubes to coat them evenly and allow them to sit for 10 minutes.
4. Add the sesame oil to a large wok pan and heat it over medium-high heat.
5. Stir in the garlic, followed by the tofu cubes; stir-fry while continuously stirring to prevent burning.
6. Add the Chinese cabbage and shallots and stir-fry all ingredients for another minute.
7. Next, add the zoodles with the remaining sauce and the water. Allow the mixture to cook for another minute.
8. Finally add the bean sprouts, toss the ingredients, and turn off the heat.
9. Serve (with the optional julienned carrots on top, if desired), and enjoy!
10. Alternatively, store the zoodles and tofu mixture separately in the fridge using a 2-compartment airtight container. Consume within 4 days.

*Tip: Use more tofu or serve the dish with a fried egg for an ovo-version with more protein!*

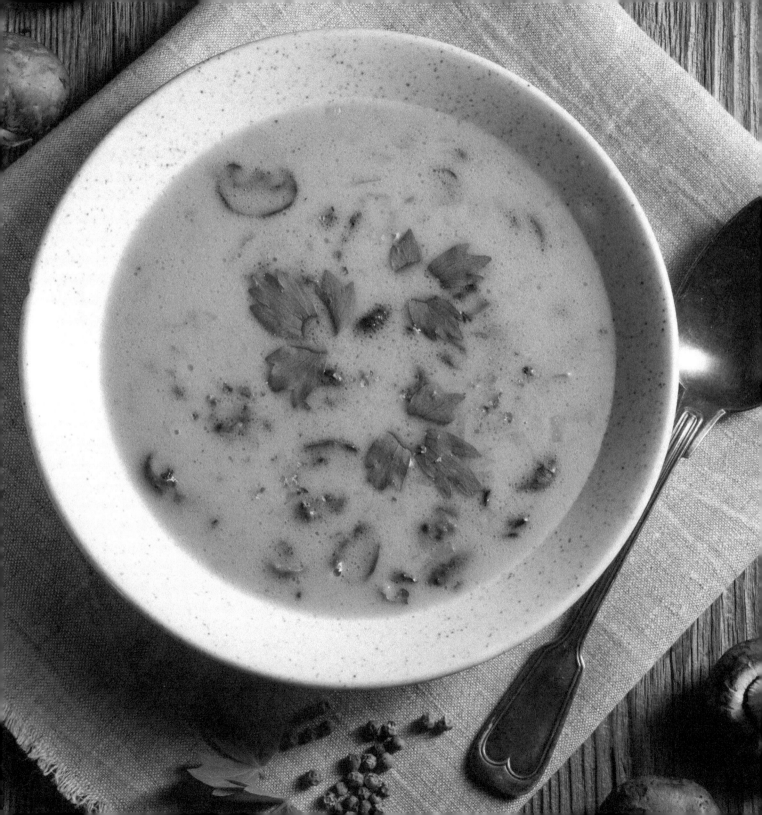

# 7. Tofu Setan ⊗

Serves: 2 | Prep Time: ~15 min |

**Nutrition Information**
(per serving)
- Calories: 311 kcal
- Net Carbs: 6.7 g.
- Fat: 23.45 g.
- Protein: 17.9 g.
- Fiber: 3.1 g.
- Sugar: 4.95 g.

## INGREDIENTS:
- 1 12-oz. pack extra firm tofu (drained, cubed)
- 2 tbsp. coconut oil
- 2 garlic cloves
- 1 medium onion (chopped)
- 2 red chilis (finely chopped, more to taste)
- 2 tbsp. soy sauce
- 1½ tbsp. low-carb maple syrup
- ½ tbsp. mustard
- ¼ cup water
- Optional: ¼ cup spring onions (finely chopped)

Total number of ingredients: 10

## METHOD:

1. Take a large skillet and put it over medium-high heat.
2. Add the coconut oil and tofu cubes, stirring occasionally, until the tofu starts to brown.
3. Meanwhile, in a blender or food processor, add the garlic, onions, chilis, soy sauce, maple syrup, and mustard; process the ingredients into a rough paste.
4. Add the paste to the skillet and stir for about a minute or until the paste starts to caramelize.
5. Add the water to the skillet and turn the heat down to medium.
6. Let the tofu setan cook while occasionally stirring, until most of the water has evaporated.
7. Take the skillet off the heat and allow the tofu setan to cool down for a minute.
8. Garnish with the optional spring onions if desired, serve, and enjoy!
9. Alternatively, store the tofu setan in an airtight container in the fridge. Consume within 3 days. Store in the freezer for a maximum of 30 days and thaw at room temperature. Use a microwave, toaster oven, or frying pan to reheat the tofu setan.

*Tip: Serve with cauliflower rice and pickled vegetables for an authentic low-carb Asian dish.*

# 8. Tofu Rendang ⑱

Serves: 2 | Prep Time: ~20 min |

**Nutrition Information**
(per serving)
- Calories: 331 kcal
- Net Carbs: 9.9 g.
- Fat: 27.8 g.
- Protein: 9 g.
- Fiber: 3.8 g.
- Sugar: 4.2 g.

## INGREDIENTS:
- 1 12-oz. pack extra firm tofu (drained, cubed)
- 4 tbsp. MCT oil
- 1 cinnamon stick
- 3 cloves
- 1 stalk lemon grass (white part removed)
- 3 star anise
- 3 cardamom pods
- ½ cup coconut cream
- ¼ cup water
- 1 tbsp. low-carb maple syrup
- 5 kaffir lime leaves (bruised)
- ¼ cup toasted coconut flakes

*Spice Paste:*
- 6 shallots
- 2-inch piece ginger
- 3 stalks lemon grass (only white parts)
- 3 garlic cloves
- 5 dried red chilis (more or less to taste)

Total number of ingredients: 17

## METHOD:

1. Add the spice paste ingredients to a blender and process them into a fine paste.
2. Take a large skillet, put it over medium-high heat, and add the MCT oil.
3. Add the spice paste, cinnamon, cloves, star anise, and cardamom pods to the skillet.
4. Stir-fry the ingredients until the spices become aromatic.
5. Add the lemon grass and tofu cubes to the skillet; make sure to incorporate all ingredients.
6. Add the coconut cream, maple syrup, and water to skillet. Stir again until all ingredients are fully incorporated; then turn the heat down to medium.
7. Add the kaffir lime leaves and toasted coconut flakes. Stir to make sure all ingredients combine.
8. Let the tofu rendang cook while occasionally stirring, until most of the water has evaporated.
9. Take the skillet off the heat, serve and enjoy!
10. Alternatively, store the tofu rendang in an airtight container in the fridge. Consume within 3 days. Store in the freezer for a maximum of 30 days, and thaw at room temperature. Use a microwave, toaster oven, or skillet to reheat the tofu rendang.

*Note: Cooking vastly reduces the heat of the chilis since the capsaicin oils spread out through the entire dish and become less concentrated.*

*Tip: Serve the dish with cauliflower rice and pickled vegetables for an authentic low-carb Asian dish.*

# 9. Moo Goo Gai Pan ⑧

Serves: 2 | Prep Time: ~20 min |

**Nutrition Information**
(per serving)
- Calories: 323 kcal
- Net Carbs: 7.8 g.
- Fat: 24.8 g.
- Protein: 16.2 g.
- Fiber: 4 g.
- Sugar: 5.6 g.

## INGREDIENTS:
- 1 12-oz. pack extra firm tofu
  (drained, cubed)
- 2 tbsp. coconut oil
- ½ cup carrots (julienned
  or thinly sliced)
- 2 cups mushrooms (sliced)
- 1 cup bamboo shoots
- 1 tbsp. water
- 2 garlic cloves (minced)
- 1-inch piece ginger (finely minced)
- Salt and pepper to taste

*Sauce:*
- 1 cup vegetable broth (page 29)
- 1 tbsp. low-carb maple syrup
- 1 tbsp. low-sodium soy sauce
- 1 tbsp. sesame oil
- 1 tsp. agar agar

Total number of ingredients: 15

## METHOD:

1. Take a large skillet, put it over medium-high heat and add 1 tablespoon of the coconut oil.
2. Add the carrots and a tablespoon of water. Cook the carrots for 3 minutes while stirring.
3. Add in the mushrooms and cook until the slices are lightly brown and tender.
4. Stir in the bamboo shoots and cook all ingredients for about a minute. Add salt and pepper to taste.
5. Remove the vegetables from the skillet, transfer them onto a plate, and cover with foil to keep the veggies warm.
6. In a small bowl, mix the sauce ingredients. Stir well and set the sauce aside.
7. Wipe the skillet with a paper towel to remove any excess liquid and add the remaining tablespoon of coconut oil to the skillet.
8. Add the tofu cubes to the skillet and stir while seasoning the tofu cubes with salt and pepper to taste.
9. Continue to add the ginger and garlic to the skillet. Allow the ingredients to cook for about a minute.
10. Add the vegetables back into the skillet, heat them through for a minute, and then pour in the previously made sauce.
11. Turn heat up to high and wait until the sauce begins to boil. Allow it to cook for a minute while occasionally stirring.
12. Take the skillet of the heat, serve, and enjoy!
13. Alternatively, store the moo goo gai pan in an airtight container in the fridge. Consume within 3 days. Store in the freezer for a maximum of 30 days, and thaw at room temperature. Use a microwave, toaster oven or skillet to reheat the moo goo gai pan.

*Tip: Serve with cauliflower rice or shirataki noodles!*

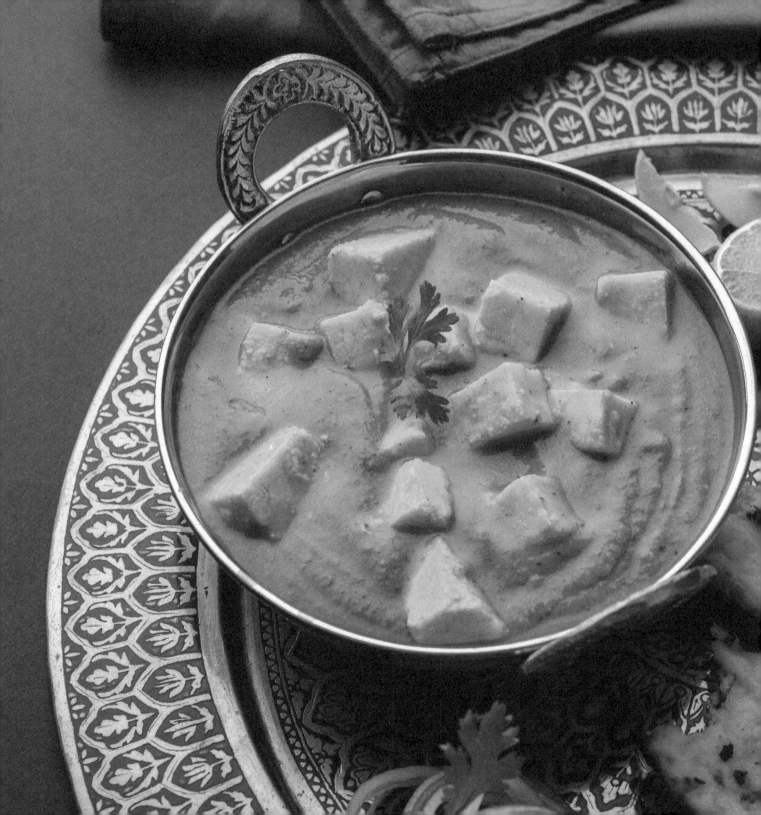

# 10. Palek Tofu Curry ⊛

Serves: 4 | Prep Time: ~30 min |

## Nutrition Information
(per serving)
- Calories: 196 kcal
- Net Carbs: 7.7 g.
- Fat: 12 g.
- Protein: 13.3 g.
- Fiber: 6.4 g.
- Sugar: 3.7 g.

## INGREDIENTS:
- 1 12-oz. pack extra firm tofu (drained, cubed)
- 6 cups fresh spinach (rinsed, drained)
- 1 green chili (seeded, chopped)
- ½-inch piece ginger (chopped)
- 1 small onion (finely chopped)
- 1 medium tomato (cubed)
- 4 garlic cloves (minced)
- ½ tsp. cumin seeds
- ½ tsp. red chili powder
- 1 tsp. turmeric powder
- 1 tsp. garam masala powder
- 1 bay leaf
- ½ cup water
- 2 tbsp. coconut cream
- 2 tbsp. MCT oil
- Salt to taste
- Optional: 4 lemon wedges

Total number of ingredients: 17

## METHOD:

1. In a food processor or blender, add the spinach leaves, green chilis, and ginger. Blend until a smooth paste-like substance forms and set this aside.
2. Put a large skillet over medium heat and add the MCT oil.
3. Add the cumin seeds, bay leaf, and onions to the skillet while stirring.
4. Sauté the onions until browned; then add the garlic and give the ingredients a stir.
5. Add the tomato cubes and keep stirring until these have softened.
6. Once the tomato cubes are soft, add the red chili powder and turmeric powder and mix thoroughly.
7. Add the spinach mixture to the skillet and mix well, until it is fully incorporated.
8. Add the ½ cup of water to the skillet, stir, and lower the heat to a simmer.
9. Cover the skillet and allow the curry to simmer for about 5 minutes.
10. Stir in the garam masala powder before adding the tofu cubes to the skillet. Stir carefully and let the curry simmer for another 5 minutes.
11. Stir in the coconut cream and stir gently to make sure the cream fully blends with the curry.
12. Take the skillet off the heat and allow the curry to cool down for a minute.
13. Serve the curry, garnished with the optional lemon wedges if desired, and enjoy!
14. Alternatively, store the curry in an airtight container in the fridge. Consume within 3 days. Store in the freezer for a maximum of 30 days, and thaw at room temperature. Use a microwave or saucepan to reheat the palek tofu curry.

# 11. Tom Yum Soup ⓥ

**Nutrition Information**
(per serving)
- Calories: 130 kcal
- Net Carbs: 7 g.
- Fat: 7.4 g.
- Protein: 9.7 g.
- Fiber: 2.7 g.
- Sugar: 2.9 g.

## INGREDIENTS:
- 1 12-oz. pack extra firm tofu (drained, cubed)
- 6 cups vegetable broth (page 29)
- 1 stalk lemon grass (white part removed, finely minced)
- 3 garlic cloves (finely minced)
- 1 medium onion (finely chopped)
- 1-inch piece ginger (finely chopped)
- 3 kaffir lime leaves (bruised)
- 1 tsp. lime juice
- ½ tbsp. soy sauce
- 1 cup shiitake mushrooms (sliced)
- 1 cup cherry tomatoes (halved)
- ¼ cup coconut cream
- Optional: 1 tsp. chili oil (more to taste)
- Optional: ¼ cup cilantro (chopped)

Total number of ingredients: 14

## METHOD:
1. Put a large cooking pot over high heat and add the vegetable broth.
2. Add the lemon grass and let the broth boil for about 5 minutes.
3. Stir in the garlic, onions, ginger, kaffir lime leaves, lime juice, and soy sauce.
4. Turn the heat down to medium-high, cover the pot, and let the soup softly boil for another 5 minutes.
5. Add the mushrooms to the pot and let the soup cook for another 5 minutes while occasionally stirring.
6. Add the tofu cubes and cherry tomatoes, cook for another 2 minutes, and then stir in the coconut cream.
7. Bring the heat down to medium, add the optional chili oil to taste, if desired, and stir.
8. Take the pot off the heat and allow the soup to cool down for a few minutes.
9. Serve warm, garnish with the optional cilantro if desired, and enjoy.
10. Alternatively, store the soup in an airtight container in the fridge. Consume within 3 days. Store each serving individually in the freezer for a maximum of 30 days, and thaw at room temperature. Use a microwave or pot to reheat the soup.

# 12. Stuffed Zucchini ⊕

Serves: 2 | Prep Time: ~20 min |

**Nutrition Information**
(per serving)
- Calories: 359.5 kcal
- Net Carbs: 8.75 g.
- Fat: 32.5 g.
- Protein: 7.3 g.
- Fiber: 4.3 g.
- Sugar: 6.3 g.

## INGREDIENTS:
- 1 large zucchini
- 2 tbsp. olive oil
- ¼ cup green onion (chopped)
- 1 garlic clove (minced)
- 1 cup fresh baby spinach leaves
- Handful of fresh rocket (chopped)
- Sea salt and black pepper to taste
- ¼ cup vegan cheese (page 79)
- Pinch of dried parsley

Total number of ingredients: 10

## METHOD:

1. Preheat the oven to 375°F/190°C and line a baking tray with parchment paper.
2. Cut the zucchini in half lengthwise and scoop out most of the pulp.
3. Mash the zucchini pulp in a small bowl with a masher and set it aside.
4. Heat a large skillet over medium heat and add half of the olive oil.
5. Add the zucchini pulp, chopped onion, and minced garlic to the skillet.
6. Stir continuously, cooking the ingredients for up to 5 minutes before adding the baby spinach and rocket.
7. Stir for a few seconds, season with salt and pepper to taste, and turn off the heat.
8. Add the vegan cheese and stir well to ensure all ingredients are incorporated and the cheese has melted.
9. Scoop the mixture into the zucchini halves and transfer them onto the baking tray.
10. Cover the baking tray with aluminum foil and transfer it to the oven.
11. Bake the stuffed zucchini halves for 25 minutes. Then, turn off the oven, uncover the baking tray, and put the uncovered zucchini halves back into the oven for a few more minutes.
12. Serve the stuffed zucchini garnished with the remaining olive oil and some dried parsley.
13. Serve and enjoy!
14. Alternatively, store the stuffed zucchini in an airtight container in the fridge and consume within 3 days. Store in the freezer for a maximum of 30 days and thaw at room temperature. Reheat in the microwave for about 40-60 seconds.

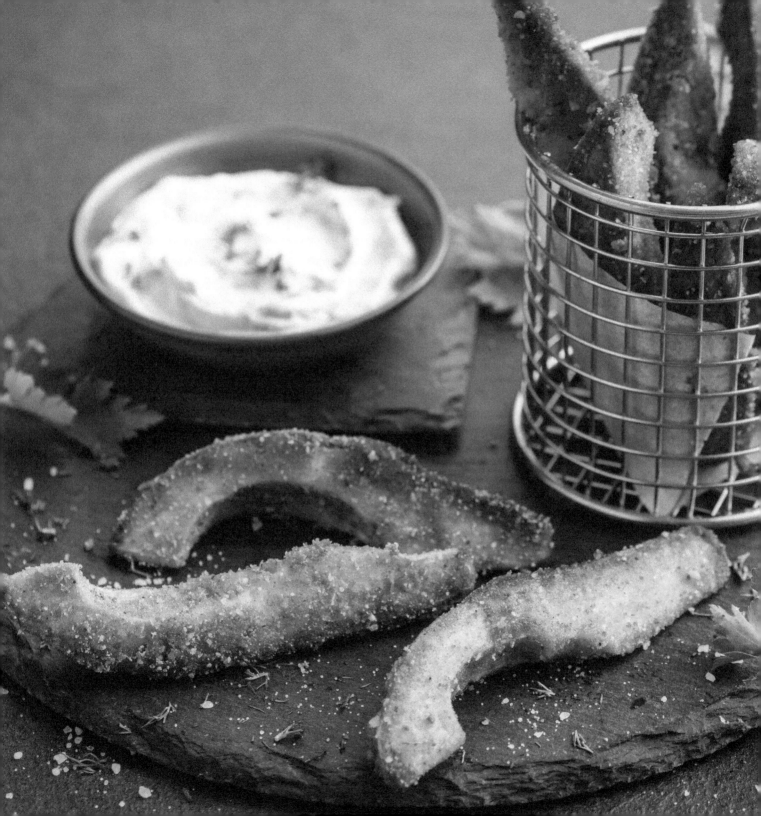

# 13. Avocado Fries ⊚

Serves: 2 | Prep Time: ~30 min |

## Nutrition Information
(per serving)
- Calories: 333.7 kcal
- Net Carbs: 3.3 g.
- Fat: 31.9 g.
- Protein: 7 g.
- Fiber: 8.1 g.
- Sugar: 3.05 g.

## INGREDIENTS:
- 1 tbsp. olive oil
- ½ cup almond flour
- ¼ tsp. cayenne pepper
- ¼ tsp. smoked paprika
- Pinch of salt
- ¾ tbsp. unsweetened almond milk
- 1 medium Hass avocado (pitted, peeled)
- 1 tsp. lime juice

Total number of ingredients: 8

## METHOD:

1. Preheat the oven to 400°F/200°C.
2. Line a baking tray with parchment paper and grease the paper with the olive oil.
3. In a small bowl, combine the flour, cayenne pepper, smoked paprika, and salt.
4. Pour the almond milk into another small bowl.
5. Slice the peeled avocado into 10 equally-sized fries.
6. Coat all sides of the fries in the flour mixture, dip in almond milk, and coat with another layer of flour.
7. Transfer the coated fries to the greased baking tray.
8. Bake the fries for 5 minutes, then flip them over and bake for another 10 minutes. Flip the fries again and bake for 5 more minutes.
9. Flip the fries one more time, sprinkle them with the lime juice, and bake them for a final 5 minutes.
10. Take the baking tray out of the oven and allow the fries to cool down for a few minutes.
11. Serve warm with any low-carb (vegan) sauce and enjoy!
12. Alternatively, store the avocado fries in an airtight container in the fridge and consume within 2 days. Store in the freezer for a maximum of 30 days and thaw at room temperature. Reheat in the microwave for about 40-60 seconds.

# 14. Mushroom Zoodle Pasta ⊚

**Nutrition Information**
(per serving)
- Calories: 421.6 kcal
- Net Carbs: 14.25 g.
- Fat: 34.9 g.
- Protein: 11.5 g.
- Fiber: 7 g.
- Sugar: 8 g.

## INGREDIENTS:
- 3 large zucchinis (spiralized into zoodles or sliced lengthwise very thinly)
- ½ tsp. salt
- 1 tbsp. coconut oil
- 1 large green onion (diced)
- 3 garlic cloves (minced)
- 5 cups oyster mushrooms (chopped)
- Pinch each of nutmeg, onion powder, paprika powder, white pepper, and salt
- 1 cup full-fat coconut milk
- ½ cup vegan mozzarella (page 79)
- ½ cup baby spinach leaves (chopped)
- ¼ cup fresh thyme (chopped)
- Optional: 1 tbsp. miso paste

Total number of ingredients: 14

## METHOD:

1. In a large bowl, toss the zoodles or zucchini slices with half a teaspoon of salt and set aside.
2. Put a large skillet, over medium heat and add the coconut oil.
3. Add the onion and cook until translucent, for about 5 minutes while stirring occasionally.
4. Stir in the minced garlic, chopped mushrooms, and remaining seasonings.
5. Cook all ingredients in the skillet for about 3 minutes, stirring continuously.
6. Reduce heat to medium-low and slowly incorporate the coconut milk, followed by the mozzarella.
7. Cover the skillet and let the ingredients heat through for about 8 minutes, stirring occasionally.
8. Drain any excess liquid from the salted zoodles by dabbing them with paper towels.
9. Add the dry zoodles to the skillet with the chopped spinach and stir well until all ingredients are combined.
10. Turn off the heat and top the mushroom zoodle pasta with the chopped thyme.
11. Add more seasonings to taste, serve the pasta in a bowl, and enjoy!
12. Alternatively, store the pasta in an airtight container in the fridge and consume within 4 days. Store for a maximum of 60 days in the freezer and thaw at room temperature. Reheat in the microwave for about 1 minute.

# 15. Quick Veggie Protein Bowl ⑧

Serves: 1 | Prep Time: ~18 min |

**Nutrition Information**
(per serving)
- Calories: 296 kcal
- Net Carbs: 7.75 g.
- Fat: 20.95 g.
- Protein: 17.8 g.
- Fiber: 8.15 g.
- Sugar: 3.35 g.

## INGREDIENTS:
- 4 oz. extra-firm tofu (drained)
- ¼ tsp. turmeric
- ¼ tsp. cayenne pepper
- 1 tbsp. coconut oil
- 1 cup broccoli florets (diced)
- 1 cup Chinese kale (diced)
- ½ cup button mushrooms (diced)
- ½ tsp. dried oregano
- Himalayan salt and ground black pepper to taste
- ½ tsp. paprika
- Optional: ¼ cup of fresh oregano (diced)

Total number of ingredients: 12

## METHOD:

1. Cut the tofu into tiny pieces and season with the turmeric and cayenne pepper.
2. Warm a large skillet over medium heat and add ¾ of the coconut oil.
3. Once oil is heated, add the tofu and cook it for about 5 minutes, stirring continuously.
4. Transfer the cooked tofu to a medium-sized bowl and set it aside.
5. Add the remaining coconut oil, diced broccoli florets, Chinese kale, button mushrooms, and the remaining herbs to the skillet. Season with the salt, pepper, and paprika to taste.
6. Cook the vegetables for 6-8 minutes, stirring continuously.
7. Turn off the heat and transfer the cooked veggies and tofu to the bowl. Garnish with the optional fresh oregano.
8. Serve and enjoy!
9. Alternatively, store the quick veggie protein bowl in an airtight container in the fridge and consume within 4 days. Store for a maximum of 60 days in the freezer and thaw at room temperature before serving.

# 16. Vizza ⊚

Serves: 3 | Prep Time: ~40 min |

**Nutrition Information**
(per serving)
- Calories: 360.9 kcal
- Net Carbs: 10 g.
- Fat: 28.85 g.
- Protein: 13.5 g.
- Fiber: 11.5 g.
- Sugar: 5.5 g.

## INGREDIENTS:

*Crust:*
- 16 oz. cauliflower rice
  (or, pulse 4 ½ cups stemless
  cauliflower florets into rice)
- 3 flax eggs (page 27)
- 2 tbsp. chia seeds
- ½ cup almond flour
- ½ tsp. garlic powder
- ½ tsp. dried basil
- Pinch of salt
- Optional: 2 tsp. water

*Topping:*
- ½ cup simple marinara sauce
  (page 28)
- 1 medium zucchini (sliced)
- 1 medium green bell pepper
  (pitted, cored, sliced)
- 1 cup button mushrooms (diced)
- ½ cup vegan cheese (page 79)
- Sea salt and ground black
  pepper to taste
- Optional: 1 jalapeño pepper
  (pitted, cored, diced)
- Optional: pinch of cayenne pepper
- Optional: handful of fresh rocket

Total number of ingredients: 17

## METHOD:

1. Preheat the oven to 400°F/200°C and line a baking sheet with parchment paper.
2. Transfer the cauliflower rice to a large saucepan and add enough water to cover the 'rice.' Bring the water to a soft boil over medium heat. Cover the saucepan, turn down the heat to medium-low, and allow the rice to simmer for about 5 minutes before draining the water off. This step can be skipped if store-bought cauliflower rice is used.
3. Transfer the cauliflower rice onto a clean dish towel and close the cloth by holding the edges. Wring out any excess water by twisting the lower part of the towel that contains the rice.
4. Once the cauliflower rice is completely drained, transfer the towel to the freezer for up to 15 minutes. Doing so will cool the rice.
5. When the cauliflower rice has cooled completely, put it into a large bowl.
6. Add the flax eggs, chia seeds, almond flour, garlic, dried basil, and salt. Combine all the ingredients into a firm, kneadable dough. If the dough is too firm, add the optional 2 tablespoons of water.
7. Spread the dough over the entire surface of the baking dish. The uncooked crust should be about ¼-inch thick.
8. Bake the crust in the oven for 25 minutes, then sprinkle some additional water on top and bake for another 5 minutes. The top of the crust will turn lightly golden.
9. Take the baking tray out of the oven and allow the crust to cool for a few minutes.
10. Spread the marinara sauce evenly over the golden crust. Do the same for the vegetables.
11. Finally, garnish the vizza with the vegan cheese, optional jalapeño, and cayenne pepper.
12. Season the vizza with salt and pepper and transfer it back into the oven for a few more minutes.
13. Serve the vizza warm, garnished with a handful of fresh rocket, and enjoy!
14. Alternatively, store vizza slices in an airtight container in the fridge and consume within 4 days. Store for a maximum of 60 days in the freezer and thaw at room temperature. Reheat in a toaster oven for about 5 minutes.

*Tip: Fancy a spicy bite? Be sure to use the optional topping ingredients!*

# 17. Tofu Cheeze Nuggets & Zucchini Fries

**Serves: 2 | Prep Time: ~40 min |**

## Nutrition Information
(per serving)
- Calories: 813.5 kcal
- Net Carbs: 9 g.
- Fat: 72.1 g.
- Protein: 30.35 g.
- Fiber: 10.7 g.
- Sugar: 7.9 g.

## INGREDIENTS:

*Tofu Cheese Nuggets:*
- 1 (12 oz. pack) extra firm tofu (drained, cubed)
- ½ cup smoked chipotle cream cheese (page 85)
- ½ cup almond flour
- 2 tbsp. water

*Zucchini Fries:*
- 2 tsp. red chili flakes
- ½ cup almond flour
- ¼ cup olive oil
- 1 large zucchini (skinned, cut into sticks)

Total number of ingredients: 8

## METHOD:

1. Preheat the oven to 400°F/200°C and line a baking tray with parchment paper.
2. Put the cream cheese, ½ cup almond flour, and water into a large bowl and mix thoroughly until all the ingredients are combined.
3. Add the tofu cubes to the bowl and coat all the cubes evenly.
4. Transfer the coated tofu cubes onto one half of the baking tray and set it aside.
5. Put the chili flakes and almond flour into a large bowl and mix until all ingredients are combined.
6. Pour the olive oil into a medium-sized bowl and dip each zucchini stick into the oil. Make sure to cover all fries evenly.
7. Put the zucchini fries in the bowl with the almond flour mixture and gently stir the fries around until they are all evenly covered.
8. Transfer the zucchini fries onto the baking tray with the tofu nuggets and spread them out evenly. If the nuggets and fries don't fit on the baking tray together, bake them in two batches.
9. Put the baking tray into the oven and bake the nuggets and fries for about 18 minutes, or until golden-brown and crispy.
10. Take the baking tray out of the oven and let the dish cool down for about a minute.
11. Serve and enjoy with a light salad of greens as a side dish.
12. Alternatively, store the tofu nuggets and zucchini fries in an airtight container in the fridge and consume within 3 days. Store in the freezer for a maximum of 30 days and thaw at room temperature. Use a toaster oven or skillet to reheat the tofu nuggets and zucchini fries.

# 18. Avocado Spring Rolls

**Nutrition Information**
(per serving)
- Calories: 503 kcal
- Net Carbs: 12.4 g.
- Fat: 45 g.
- Protein: 10 g.
- Fiber: 11.6 g.
- Sugar: 7.5 g.

## INGREDIENTS:
- 2 medium Hass avocados (peeled, pitted, sliced)
- 1-inch piece ginger (grated)
- 1 garlic clove (minced)
- Juice of ½ lemon
- ½ cup cabbage (shredded)
- ¼ cup carrots (julienned or matchsticks)
- 4-6 coconut wraps
- 2 tbsp. olive oil

*Spicy Almond Sauce:*
- ½ cup almond butter
- 2 tsp. low-sodium soy sauce
- ½ tsp. rice vinegar
- Juice of ½ lemon
- ½ tsp. chili garlic paste (page 31)
- 1 tbsp. low-carb maple syrup
- 2 tsp. sesame oil

Total number of ingredients: 14

## METHOD:

1. In a small bowl, gently toss together the sliced avocado, ginger, garlic, lemon juice, cabbage, and julienned carrots.
2. Put a coconut wrap on a flat and dry surface. Place about ¼ of the avocado mixture in the center of the wrap.
3. Fold the wrap about ½ inch inward on two parallel sides and roll the wrap up until the mixture is covered.
4. Repeat with the remaining 3-5 wraps until all of the avocado mixture is used.
5. Put a skillet over medium-high heat and warm the olive oil until shimmering.
6. Add the spring rolls to the skillet and brown them, about 30 seconds on each side.
7. Prepare the sauce by putting all the sauce ingredients into a medium-sized bowl and stir thoroughly. Add one or more tablespoon of warm water, if necessary, to achieve the desired consistency.
8. Serve the spring rolls warm with the spicy almond sauce as a dip and enjoy!
9. Alternatively, store the spring rolls and sauce separately in an airtight container in the fridge, and consume within 2 days. Store in the freezer for a maximum of 30 days and thaw at room temperature. Use a microwave, toaster oven, or frying pan to reheat the spring rolls.

*Note: Most of the net carbs in this recipe come from the coconut wraps, using a wrap with lower carbs might be a better fit for carb restriction.*

# 19. Cauliflower Curry Soup ⑧

Serves: 4 | Prep Time: ~45 min |

**Nutrition Information**
(per serving)
- Calories: 390.5 kcal
- Net Carbs: 7.46 g.
- Fat: 34.2 g.
- Protein: 12.25 g.
- Fiber: 5.61 g.
- Sugar: 5.5 g.

## INGREDIENTS:
- 1 large cauliflower (chopped)
- 4 tbsp. olive oil
- ½ red onion (finely chopped)
- 4 garlic cloves (minced)
- 1 tbsp. yellow curry paste
- 1-inch piece ginger (grated)
- 1 (12 oz. pack) extra firm tofu
  (drained, scrambled)
- 1 tsp. chili flakes
- Juice of 1 medium lime
- 4 cups vegetable broth (page 29)
- 1 tbsp. sesame oil
- 1 tsp. low-sodium soy sauce
- 1 cup full-fat coconut milk

Total number of ingredients: 13

## METHOD:

1. Preheat the oven to 400°F/200°C and line a baking tray with parchment paper.
2. Put the cauliflower florets on the baking tray and drizzle 2 tablespoons of olive oil over them, covering them evenly.
3. Put the baking tray into the oven and bake for about 25-30 minutes, until the florets are golden brown.
4. Put a large pot over medium heat and add the remaining 2 tablespoons of olive oil.
5. Take the baking tray out of the oven and set it aside for a few minutes to let the cauliflower florets cool down.
6. Add the onion and garlic to the pot and fry for about a minute, stirring occasionally.
7. Add the curry paste to the pot along with the ginger, scrambled tofu, and chili flakes. Stir for another minute.
8. Put the baked cauliflower florets into a blender or food processor, along with the vegetable broth, sesame oil, soy sauce, and coconut milk.
9. Blend these ingredients until smooth, then transfer the mixture into the pot.
10. Incorporate all the ingredients, stirring occasionally until the contents of the pot start to cook. Once the soup reaches the boiling point, bring the heat down to a simmer.
11. Cover the pot and let the soup simmer for about 10 minutes, then take the pot off the heat and set it aside to cool for a few minutes.
12. Divide the soup between 2 medium-sized bowls, serve and enjoy!
13. Alternatively, store the cauliflower curry soup in an airtight container in the fridge and consume within 3 days. Store in the freezer for a maximum of 30 days and thaw at room temperature. Use a microwave or pot to reheat the cauliflower soup.

# 20. Cashew Siam Stir-Fry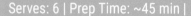

Serves: 6 | Prep Time: ~45 min |

**Nutrition Information**
(per serving)
- Calories: 160 kcal
- Net Carbs: 5.9 g.
- Fat: 11.9 g.
- Protein: 7 g.
- Fiber: 1.6 g.
- Sugar: 2 g.

## INGREDIENTS:
- 2 tbsp. olive oil
- ½ cup raw cashews (unsalted)
- ½ green onion (finely chopped)
- 4 garlic cloves (minced)
- 1-inch piece ginger (grated)
- 1 red bell pepper (seeded, chopped)
- 1 (10 oz. pack) extra firm tofu (drained, cubed)
- 1 tsp. chili flakes

*Sauce:*
- 1 tbsp. low-sodium soy sauce
- 3 tsp. rice vinegar
- 1 tbsp. low-carb maple syrup
- ¼ cup vegetable broth (page 29, or use water)
- 1 tsp. sesame oil

Total number of ingredients: 13

## METHOD:
1. Put the olive oil in a large skillet over medium heat.
2. Add the cashews to the skillet and stir fry for 2 minutes.
3. Stir the chopped onion and garlic into the skillet. Keep stirring while cooking until the onion is translucent. This should take about two minutes.
4. Add the ginger and chopped bell pepper. Increase the heat to medium-high and cook the ingredients for about 3 minutes while stirring.
5. Add the tofu cubes and chili flakes. Cook for another 3 minutes, stirring occasionally.
6. Mix the sauce ingredients in a medium-sized bowl until no lumps remain and add it to the skillet.
7. Stir and cook all ingredients together for another minute, then bring the heat down to a simmer while stirring occasionally until the sauce starts to thicken.
8. Take the skillet off the heat, divide the cashew stir-fry between 2 bowls, serve and enjoy!
9. Alternatively, store the cashew stir-fry in an airtight container in the fridge and consume within 3 days. Store in the freezer for a maximum of 30 days and thaw at room temperature. Use a microwave or pot to reheat the cashew stir-fry.

# 1. No-Carb Cereal Bars ⊚

Serves: 16 bars | Prep Time: ~30 min |

## Nutrition Information
(per serving)
- Calories: 223 kcal
- Net Carbs: 2.4 g.
- Fat: 20.3 g.
- Protein: 7.2 g.
- Fiber: 3 g.
- Sugar: 0.8 g.

## INGREDIENTS:
- 1 cup pumpkin seeds
- 1 cup sunflower seeds
- 1 cup almonds
- 1 cup hazelnuts (chopped)
- 1 flax egg (page 27)
- ¼ cup almond butter
- ¼ cup cocoa butter
- 1 tsp. stevia powder
- Ground cinnamon to taste

Total number of ingredients: 9

## METHOD:

1. Preheat oven to 350°F/175°C, and line a shallow baking dish with parchment paper.
2. Transfer all the listed ingredients to a blender or food processor. Blend it into a chunky mixture.
3. Transfer the mixture onto the baking dish and spread it out evenly into a flat chunk on the parchment paper.
4. Bake this chunk for about 15 minutes.
5. Take the baking dish out of the oven and let cool down for about 10 minutes.
6. Cut the chunk into the desired number of bars while it's still a bit warm.
7. Enjoy right away or store in the fridge, using an airtight container, and consume within 6 days. Store each bar separately in the freezer, using Ziploc bags, for a maximum of 90 days. Thaw the bars at room temperature.

## SNACKS & DESSERTS

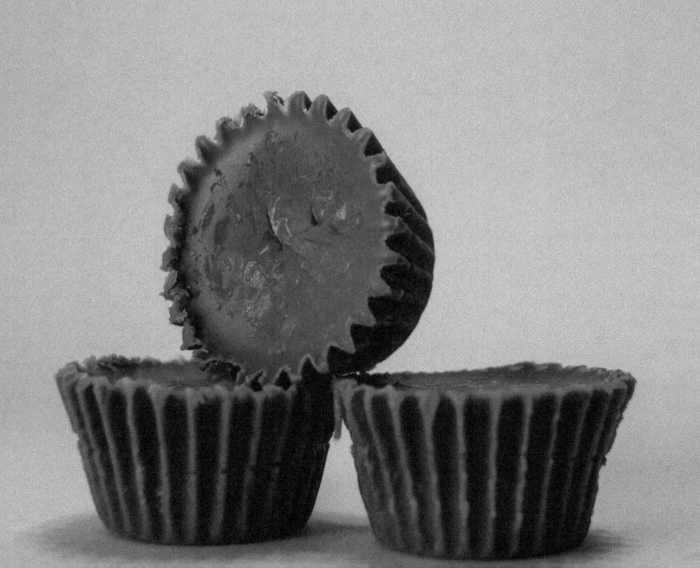

# 2. Nutty Chocolate Bombs

Serves: 12 cups | Prep Time: ~60 min |

**Nutrition Information**
(per serving)
- Calories: 253 kcal
- Net Carbs: 2.6 g.
- Fat: 24.7 g.
- Protein: 4.8 g.
- Fiber: 2.2 g.
- Sugar: 1.4 g.

## INGREDIENTS:
*Nut Butter Bottom:*
- ½ cup coconut oil
- ½ cup peanut butter (page 30)
- ½ cup almonds (chopped)
- ½ cup hazelnuts (chopped)
- ½ tbsp. pumpkin spice

*Chocolate Top:*
- ¼ cup cocoa butter
- 2 tbsp. cocoa powder
- ½ tsp. stevia powder

Total number of ingredients: 8

## METHOD:

1. Line a muffin tray with muffin liners.
2. Put the coconut oil and peanut butter in a small bowl. Heat the bowl in the microwave for 10 seconds, or until the oil and butter have melted. Make sure it doesn't get too hot.
3. Transfer the melted ingredients and the remaining nut butter bottom ingredients to a food processor or blender. Blend everything into a chunky mix.
4. Transfer 1 tablespoon of the mixture from the blender into each muffin liner.
5. Repeat this process until the blender container is empty, making sure that all 12 muffin liners are evenly filled.
6. Put the muffin tray in the freezer for about 30 minutes, until the bottom layers are firm.
7. Warm up the cocoa butter in a small saucepan over low heat until it's completely melted.
8. Stir in the cocoa powder and stevia powder. Make sure the chocolate top ingredients are well incorporated.
9. Take the muffin tray out of the freezer and divide the chocolate top mixture over the muffins. Use a teaspoon and make sure the chocolate top mixture gets evenly distributed.
10. Put the muffin tray with the covered cups back in the freezer for another 30 minutes, until the nutty chocolate bombs are firm and ready to serve.
11. Enjoy right away or store in the fridge, using an airtight container, and consume within 6 days. Store the bombs in the freezer, using Ziploc bags, for a maximum of 90 days. Thaw the bombs at room temperature.

# 3. No-Bake Hazelnut Chocolate Bars

Serves: 16 bars | Prep Time: ~60 min |

**Nutrition Information**
(per serving)
- Calories: 185 kcal
- Net Carbs: 1.8 g.
- Fat: 18 g.
- Protein: 3.4 g.
- Fiber: 2.4 g.
- Sugar: 0.8 g.

## INGREDIENTS:
- ½ cup coconut oil
- 2 cups hazelnuts
- ¼ cup almonds
- ¼ cup walnuts
- 1 tbsp. pure vanilla extract
- 1 tsp. stevia powder
- ¼ cup cocoa powder

Total number of ingredients: 7

## METHOD:

1. Line a shallow baking dish with parchment paper.
2. Transfer all the listed ingredients to a food processor or blender. Blend the ingredients into a chunky mixture.
3. Transfer the mixture onto the baking dish and spread it out evenly into a flat chunk.
4. Cover the baking dish and put it in the freezer for 45 minutes, until the chunk is firm.
5. Take the baking dish out the freezer, cut up the chunk into the desired number of bars, and store, or serve and share.
6. Enjoy right away or store in the fridge, using an airtight container and consume within 6 days. Store each bar separately in the freezer, using Ziploc bags, for a maximum of 90 days. Thaw the bars at room temperature.

# 4. Coconut Chocolate Balls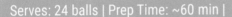

Serves: 24 balls | Prep Time: ~60 min |

**Nutrition Information**
(per serving)
- Calories: 210 kcal
- Net Carbs: 2 g.
- Fat: 20.8 g.
- Protein: 3.5 g.
- Fiber: 2.5 g.
- Sugar: 0.9 g.

## INGREDIENTS:
- ½ cup coconut oil
- 1 cup almond butter
- 1 cup macadamia nuts
- ½ cup cocoa butter
- 1 cup shredded coconut flakes
  (unsweetened)
- 6 tbsp. cocoa powder
- 1 tbsp. vanilla extract
- 1 tsp. stevia powder

Total number of ingredients: 8

## METHOD:

1. Transfer all the listed ingredients—except the shredded coconut flakes—to a food processor or blender. Blend the ingredients into a smooth mixture.

2. Line a baking tray with parchment paper to prevent the balls from sticking to the plate.

3. Scoop out a tablespoon of the chocolate and coconut mixture and roll it into a firm ball by using your hands.

4. Repeat the same for the other 23 balls. Coat each ball with the shredded coconut flakes and then transfer them to the baking tray.

5. Put the baking tray in the freezer for 45 minutes, until all balls are solid.

6. Take the baking dish out the freezer and store the coconut balls, or, serve them right away. Share the coconut chocolate balls with others and enjoy!

7. Alternatively, store the chocolate balls in the fridge, using an airtight container and consume within 6 days. Store the balls in the freezer, using Ziploc bags, for a maximum of 90 days and thaw the at room temperature.

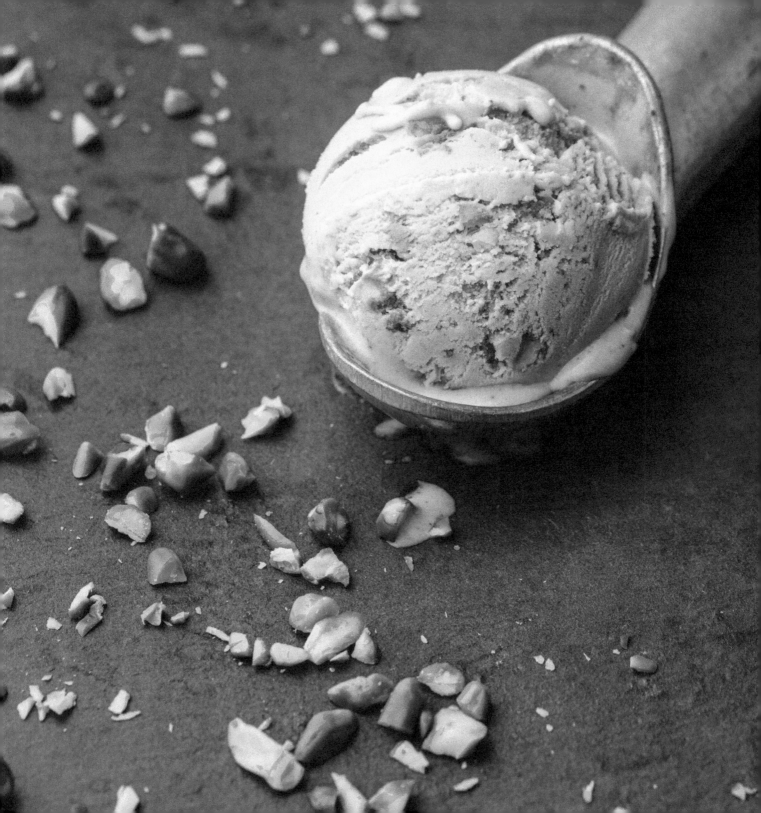

# 5. Low-Carb Pistachio Gelato

Serves: 16 | Prep Time: ~60 min |

**Nutrition Information**
(per serving)
- Calories: 212 kcal
- Net Carbs: 5.6 g.
- Fat: 19 g.
- Protein: 4.6 g.
- Fiber: 1.6 g.
- Sugar: 2 g.

## INGREDIENTS:
- 2 cups raw cashews (unsalted)
- 4 cups full-fat coconut milk
- ½ cup coconut oil
- 1½ cups pistachios
  (unsalted and shelled)
- 1 tsp. almond extract
- 2 tsp. tapioca starch
- ½ tsp. salt
- 1 tsp. stevia powder

Total number of ingredients: 8

## METHOD:

1. Cover the cashews in a small bowl filled with water, and let sit for 4 to 6 hours. Rinse and drain the cashews after soaking. Make sure no water is left.
2. Add 1 cup of pistachios to a blender or food processor, or, alternatively, use a coffee grinder; blend or grind the pistachios into a fine powder.
3. Keep or add the pistachio powder into the blender or food processor. Add the soaked nuts and the other ingredients except the remaining pistachios. Blend the ingredients into a smooth mixture.
4. Transfer the mixture to an ice cream maker and make the gelato according to the appliance's instructions. Alternatively, mix the leftover pistachios into half of the ice cream mixture and freeze it for about 4 hours. Store the other half in the fridge for this time.
5. Further blend both mixtures in the blender or food processor into the desired gelato consistency.
6. Transfer the gelato to an airtight container and put it in the freezer for about 3 hours.
7. Let the gelato thaw for 15 minutes before serving. Enjoy!
8. The pistachio gelato can be stored, using an airtight container, for a maximum of 12 months. Thaw for about 5 minutes before serving.

# 6. Raspberry Cheesecake Fudge ⊚

Serves: 12 | Prep Time: ~60 min |

**Nutrition Information**
(per serving)
- Calories: 178 kcal
- Net Carbs: 4.7 g.
- Fat: 12.7 g.
- Protein: 10.9 g.
- Fiber: 1.9 g.
- Sugar: 2.1 g.

## INGREDIENTS:
- ½ cup coconut cream
- 1 cup raw cashews (unsalted)
- ½ cup macadamia nuts (unsalted)
- ½ cup vegan protein powder (vanilla flavor)
- 2 tsp. nutritional yeast
- 2 tbsp. freeze-dried raspberry powder

Total number of ingredients: 6

## METHOD:

1. Line a deep baking dish with parchment paper.
2. Transfer all the listed ingredients to a food processor or blender. Blend the ingredients into a smooth mixture.
3. Transfer the mixture onto the deep baking dish and spread it out into an even layer.
4. Put the baking dish in the freezer for 45 minutes, until the fudge chunk is firm.
5. Take the baking dish out the freezer, cut the chunk into the desired number of fudge servings, and enjoy right away!
6. Alternatively, store the fudge in the fridge, using an airtight container, and consume within 6 days. Store in the freezer for a maximum of 90 days and thaw at room temperature.

# 7. Blueberry Lemon Choco Cups

Serves: 12 | Prep Time: ~60 min |

**Nutrition Information**
(per serving)
- Calories: 178 kcal
- Net Carbs: 1.5 g.
- Fat: 18.7 g.
- Protein: 0.8 g.
- Fiber: 1.1 g.
- Sugar: 0.4 g.

## INGREDIENTS:
- ½ cup cocoa butter
- ½ cup coconut oil
- ¼ cup cocoa powder
- 2 tbsp. organic lemon zest
- ¼ cup fresh lemon juice
- ½ tsp. stevia powder
- 20 blueberries

Total number of ingredients: 7

## METHOD:

1. Put the cocoa butter and coconut oil in a medium-sized bowl. Heat this bowl in the microwave for 10 seconds, until the butter and oil have melted. Make sure it doesn't get too hot.
2. Take the bowl out of the microwave and mix in all the remaining ingredients. Make sure everything is well incorporated.
3. Line a muffin tray with muffin liners.
4. Scoop the soft mixture out of the bowl with a tablespoon into the muffin liners. If the mixture isn't soft enough to be transferred, heat it again in the microwave for 10 seconds.
5. Fill all the muffin liners evenly, 1 tablespoon at a time.
6. Refrigerate the cups for 45 minutes, until the choco cups are firm. Take the cups out, serve and enjoy!
7. Alternatively, store the blueberry lemon cups in the fridge, using an airtight container, and consume within 6 days. Store in the freezer for a maximum of 90 days and thaw at room temperature.

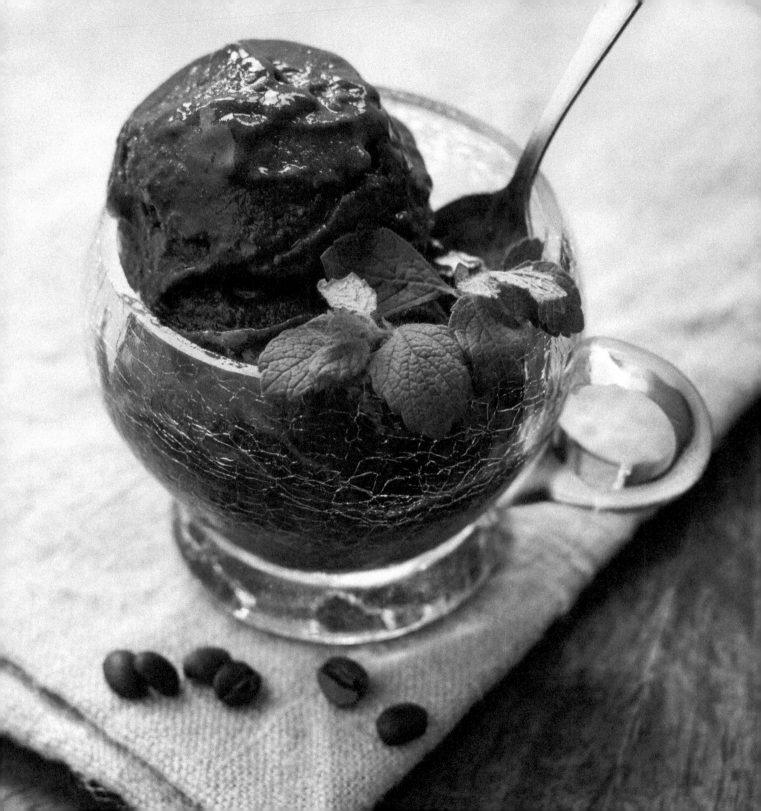

# 8. Choco Chip Ice-Cream with Mint ⊛

Serves: 8 | Prep Time: ~60 min |

**Nutrition Information**
(per serving)
- Calories: 260 kcal
- Net Carbs: 3.65 g.
- Fat: 25.7 g.
- Protein: 3.6 g.
- Fiber: 1.8 g.
- Sugar: 1.4 g.

## INGREDIENTS:
- 2 cups coconut cream
- ½ tbsp. agar-agar
- 1 ½ tbsp. water
- ¼ tsp. stevia powder (more depending on the desired sweetness)
- ½ scoop organic soy protein (chocolate flavor)
- ½ tbsp. instant coffee powder
- 1 tsp. salt
- 3 tsp. vanilla extract (more depending on desired taste)
- 4 tsp. peppermint oil (more depending on desired taste)
- 6 tbsp. dark chocolate (85% cocoa or higher, use chunks or crush a chocolate bar)
- Handful fresh mint leaves (chopped)

Total number of ingredients: 11

## METHOD:

1. Put the coconut cream in a large bowl and freeze it for at least 20 minutes.
2. Take out the cream and use a whisk to whip it for up to 10 minutes. Transfer the bowl back to the freezer.
3. In a medium-sized saucepan, add the agar-agar and water. Stir until the agar-agar has dissolved in the water, and then blend in the stevia powder.
4. Stir in the instant coffee powder and salt. Put the saucepan over medium heat. Stir constantly while heating the mixture, and make sure that no lumps remain.
5. Take the saucepan off the heat and stir in the protein powder. Set the mixture aside to cool down.
6. Take the cold coconut cream and add the vanilla extract and peppermint oil. Use more of both for a stronger taste.
7. Add the vegan gelatin mixture from the saucepan to the cream. Incorporate both mixtures by using a whisk or an electric mixer. This process is best done by working with multiple batches.
8. Taste the mixture and add more stevia, vanilla, and/or peppermint, depending on desired taste.
9. Freeze the mixture for 15 minutes. Stir it and freeze for another 10 minutes.
10. Top the ice cream with the dark chocolate chunks and freeze for at least 2 hours.
11. Allow to defrost 5 minutes before serving. Top with some additional dark chocolate, chopped mint, and enjoy!
12. The ice cream can be stored in an airtight container for a maximum of 12 months. Thaw for about 5 minutes before serving.

# 9. Creamy Coconut Vanilla Cups

**Nutrition Information**
(per serving)
- Calories: 139 kcal
- Net Carbs: 1.6 g.
- Fat: 13.5 g.
- Protein: 2.6 g.
- Fiber: 1.4 g.
- Sugar: 0.7 g.

## INGREDIENTS:
- ½ cup almond butter
- ¼ cup coconut cream
- ½ cup shredded coconut flakes (unsweetened)
- ¼ cup coconut oil
- 1 tbsp. vanilla extract
- 1 tsp. stevia powder
- Optional: 1 tsp. ground cinnamon

Total number of ingredients: 7

## METHOD:

1. Put the almond butter, coconut cream, and coconut oil in a small saucepan. Heat the pan over medium-low heat while whisking the ingredients until molten and mixed together.
2. Take the saucepan off the heat and set it aside. Let the mixture cool down.
3. Pour the mixture into a medium-sized bowl and mix in the remaining ingredients.
4. Line a muffin tray with muffin liners.
5. Scoop the soft mixture out of the bowl with a tablespoon into the muffin liners.
6. Fill all the muffin liners evenly, 1 tablespoon at a time.
7. Refrigerate the cups for 45 minutes, until the coconut cups are firm.
8. Serve and enjoy, or, store the creamy coconut vanilla cups in the fridge, using an airtight container, and consume within 6 days. Store in the freezer for a maximum of 90 days and thaw at room temperature.

# 10. Peanut Butter Power Bars

Serves: 16 | Prep Time: ~60 min |

**Nutrition Information**
(per serving)
- Calories: 178 kcal
- Net Carbs: 2 g.
- Fat: 16.8 g.
- Protein: 4.6 g.
- Fiber: 1.4 g.
- Sugar: 1.4 g.

## INGREDIENTS:
- ¼ cup almond butter
- ½ cup peanut butter (page 30)
- ½ cup coconut oil
- ¼ cup sunflower seeds
- ¼ cup walnuts (chopped)
- ¼ cup hemp seeds
- 1 tbsp. vanilla extract
- 1 tsp. stevia powder

Total number of ingredients: 8

## METHOD:

1. Put the almond butter, peanut butter, and coconut oil in a small saucepan. Heat the saucepan over medium-low heat and whisk the ingredients until everything is molten and fully incorporated.
2. Take the saucepan off the heat and set the mixture aside to cool down.
3. Line a baking dish with parchment paper.
4. Pour the contents of the saucepan into a medium-sized bowl and mix in the remaining ingredients.
5. Transfer the mixture onto the baking dish and spread it out into an even layer.
6. Put the baking dish in the freezer for 45 minutes, until the chunk is firm.
7. Take the baking dish out the freezer and cut the chunk into the desired number of bars.
8. Enjoy right away or store in the fridge, using an airtight container, and consume within 6 days. Store each bar separately in the freezer, using Ziploc bags, for a maximum of 90 days. Thaw the bars at room temperature.

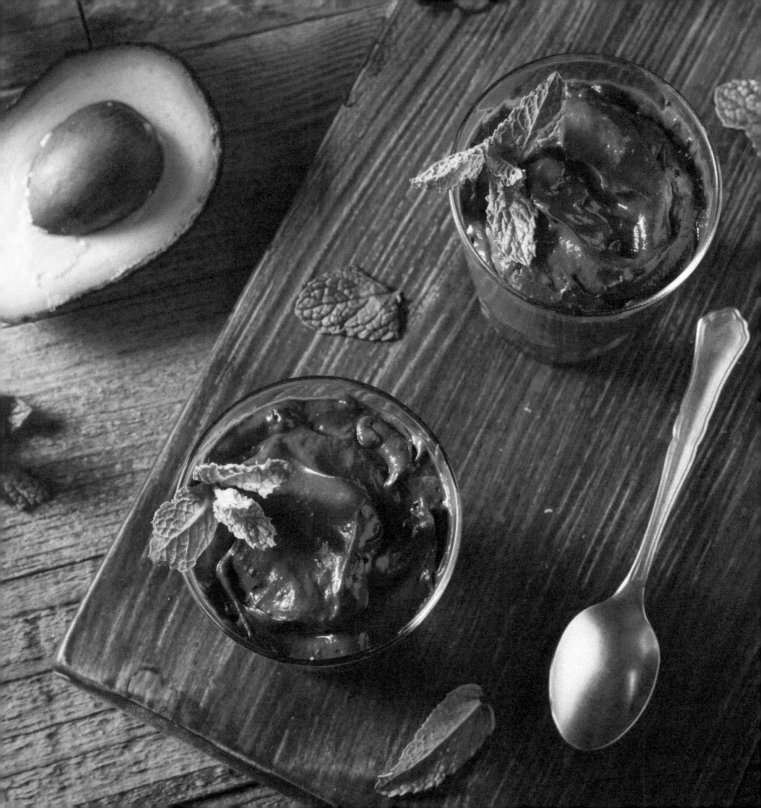

# 11. Avocado Chocolate Pudding

Serves: 4 | Prepping Time: ~10 min |

**Nutrition Information**
(per serving)
- Calories: 371 kcal
- Net Carbs: 9 g.
- Fat: 33 g.
- Protein: 7.4 g.
- Fiber: 16.7 g.
- Sugar: 4.2 g.

## INGREDIENTS:
- 4 large Hass avocados (peeled, pitted, sliced)
- ¼ cup coconut milk
- 4 tbsp. pure cocoa powder (unsweetened)
- 1 tsp. stevia sweetener
- ¼ cup dark chocolate (crushed)
- 2 tsp. vanilla extract
- 1 tsp. cinnamon powder
- Pinch of salt
- Optional: 2 tsp. lemon juice
- Optional: 2 tsp. organic lemon zest
- Optional: handful fresh mint leaves

Total number of ingredients: 11

## METHOD:

1. Add all required ingredients including the optional lemon juice and zest to a blender or food processor and blend for up to 3 minutes, until everything is combined. Scrape the sides of the blender or food processor if necessary.
2. Make sure that pudding is creamy and blend for an additional minute if necessary.
3. Transfer the pudding into one or two bowls, cover and refrigerate for at least 8 hours.
4. Serve the pudding with the optional mint leaves on top and enjoy!
5. Alternatively, store the avocado chocolate pudding in the fridge using an airtight container and consume within 2 days. 3 days when incorporating lemon juice in it.

*Tip: Top the pudding with some additional dark chocolate chips (crushed chocolate) and coconut whipped cream. Substitute the cocoa powder for chocolate soy protein!*

# 12. Dark Chocolate Mint Cups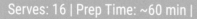

Serves: 16 | Prep Time: ~60 min |

**Nutrition Information**
(per serving)
- Calories: 151 kcal
- Net Carbs: 1.3 g.
- Fat: 15 g.
- Protein: 2.3 g.
- Fiber: 1.5 g.
- Sugar: 0.4 g.

## INGREDIENTS:
- ½ cup cocoa butter
- ½ cup almond butter
- ¼ cup coconut oil
- ¼ cup cocoa powder (unsweetened)
- 1 tsp. mint extract
- 1 tbsp. vanilla extract
- 1 tsp. stevia powder

Total number of ingredients: 7

## METHOD:

1. Put the cocoa butter, almond butter, and coconut oil in a small saucepan. Heat the pan over medium-low heat. Incorporate the ingredients using a whisk, add the cocoa powder, and whisk again until all ingredients are fully incorporated.
2. Take the saucepan off the heat and set it aside to cool down.
3. Line a baking dish with parchment paper.
4. Pour the mixture from the saucepan into a medium-sized bowl and mix in all the remaining ingredients. Make sure all ingredients are fully incorporated.
5. Transfer a tablespoon of the mixture from the bowl into each muffin liner.
6. Repeat this process until the bowl is empty, making sure that all 16 muffin liners are evenly filled.
7. Refrigerate the cups for 45 minutes, until the coconut cups are firm.
8. Take the cups out of the freezer, serve, and enjoy right away.
9. Alternatively, store the chocolate mint cups in the fridge, using an airtight container, and consume within 6 days. Store in the freezer for a maximum of 90 days and thaw at room temperature.

# 13. Toasted Cashews with Nut Flakes ⊛

Serves: 3 | Prep Time: ~20 min |

**Nutrition Information**
(per serving)
- Calories: 338 kcal
- Net Carbs: 11 g.
- Fat: 27.9 g.
- Protein: 10.3 g.
- Fiber: 2.2 g.
- Sugar: 3.7 g.

## INGREDIENTS:
- 1 cup cashews (unsalted)
- ¼ cup toasted coconut flakes
- 4 tbsp. almond flakes
- 1 tbsp. liquid monk sweetener
- ½ tbsp. cinnamon
- 4 tbsp. water
- ½ tsp. vanilla extract
- Sea salt to taste

Total number of ingredients: 8

## METHOD:

1. Put a medium-sized frying pan or skillet over medium heat.
2. Add the liquid monk sweetener, cinnamon, salt, water, and vanilla extract. Stir the ingredients until everything is combined.
3. Then add the cashew nuts while constantly stirring. Make sure to coat all the nuts evenly in the liquid mixture.
4. Keep stirring while the liquid starts to crystalize on the nuts.
5. Transfer the toasted cashews to a plate and allow them to cool down.
6. Add the toasted coconut flakes and almond flakes, and then enjoy right away.
7. Alternatively, store the nuts in the fridge, using an airtight container, and consume within 10 days.

Note: Raw coconut flakes can be toasted in the oven at 325°F/160°C for 5-10 minutes.

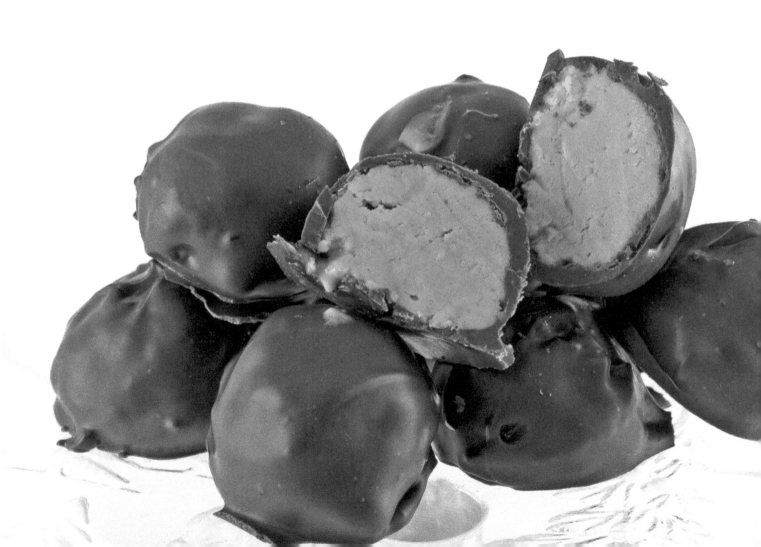

# 14. Peanut Butter Bombs

Serves: 20 | Prepping Time: ~40 min |

**Nutrition Information**
(per serving)
- Calories: 134 kcal
- Net Carbs: 4 g.
- Fat: 10.7 g.
- Protein: 5 g.
- Fiber: 2.5 g.
- Sugar: 2.6 g.

## INGREDIENTS:
- 1 cup peanut butter (page 30)
- 6 tbsp. coconut flour
- ¼ cup low-carb maple syrup
- ¼ cup organic soy protein
  (chocolate flavor)
- Optional: pinch of salt
- Optional: 1 tbsp. water
- ¾ cup dark chocolate
  (85% cocoa or higher, crushed)

Total number of ingredients: 7

## METHOD:

1. Line a large baking tray with parchment paper and set it aside.
2. In a medium-sized bowl, use a mixer to combine all the ingredients except the crushed dark chocolate. If desired, add the optional pinch of salt. Make sure all ingredients are well incorporated and no lumps remain in the batter. Add the optional water if the mixture is too thick – the batter should be spreadable.
3. Use your hands to form 20 balls and divide these over the surface of the baking tray.
4. Transfer the baking tray to the freezer and allow the balls to set for about 15 minutes.
5. Fill a small saucepan with water and put it over medium heat. Place a smaller, heat-resistant metal bowl in the water and put the crushed chocolate into it.
6. Melt the chocolate au bain-marie (in the bowl) and leave the container in the water. Be careful to keep any water from getting in the chocolate. Make sure the chocolate doesn't boil because it will ruin the flavor.
7. Take the peanut butter bombs from the freezer and roll each ball in the molten chocolate, using two forks to help you. Put each ball back onto the tray and allow the molten chocolate to firm up. Repeat this step for every peanut butter bomb.
8. Refrigerate the bombs for 15 minutes, until the chocolate layer is completely firm.
9. Serve the peanut butter bombs and enjoy!
10. Alternatively, store the bombs in the fridge using an airtight container and consume within 7 days.

# 15. Fatty Chocolate Bombs

Serves: 12 | Prepping Time: ~40 min |

**Nutrition Information**
(per serving)
- Calories: 115 kcal
- Net Carbs: 1 g.
- Fat: 11.7 g.
- Protein: 1.25 g.
- Fiber: 1.7 g.
- Sugar: 0.7 g.

## INGREDIENTS:
- ¼ cup organic soy protein (chocolate flavor)
- ½ cup coconut butter (alternatively, use almond butter)
- ¼ cup coconut oil
- ½ tsp. stevia powder
- Optional: pinch of salt
- Optional: a few fresh mint leaves

Total number of ingredients: 6

## METHOD:

1. Line a small square cake tin with parchment paper and set it aside.
2. In a medium-sized bowl, use a mixer to combine all the ingredients, including the optional salt and chopped mint leaves. Make sure all ingredients are incorporated and no lumps remain in the batter.
3. Pour the mixture into the prepared tin.
4. Transfer the cake tin to the freezer and allow the mixture to set for about 30 minutes.
5. Once set, take out the cake tin and remove the chocolate chunk. Cut it into 12 squares.
6. Serve the fatty chocolate bombs with more optional mint leaves on top and enjoy!
7. Alternatively, store the bombs in the fridge using an airtight container and consume within 7 days.

*Tip: Add some pure cocoa powder (unsweetened) and an additional teaspoon of coconut oil for a richer treat!*

# 16. Cheesecake Cups

**Nutrition Information**
(per serving)
- Calories: 217 kcal
- Net Carbs: 1.8 g.
- Fat: 21.2 g.
- Protein: 4.2 g.
- Fiber: 1.6 g.
- Sugar: 0.65 g.

## INGREDIENTS:

*Crust:*
- ½ cup pumpkin seeds (raw)
- 6 tbsp. shredded coconut (unsweetened)
- 3 tbsp. coconut oil
- 2 tbsp. organic soy protein (vanilla flavor)
- ½ tsp. stevia powder
- Pinch of salt

*Filling:*
- 6 tbsp. coconut oil
- 6 tbsp. almond butter
- 6 tbsp. coconut cream
- 2 tbsp. lemon juice
- 2 tbsp. organic soy protein (vanilla flavor)
- Pinch of salt
- Optional: ¼ tsp. xanthan gum
- Optional: ¼ tsp. stevia powder (or more to taste)

Total number of ingredients: 10

## METHOD:

1. Line a cupcake tin with 6 cupcake liners.
2. Heat a small frying pan over medium-high heat.
3. Toast the pumpkin seeds in the frying pan, stirring occasionally for about 4 minutes.
4. Add the shredded coconut and stir thoroughly to toast everything evenly.
5. Take the frying pan off the heat and allow the ingredients to cool down before transferring them into a food processor or blender. Pulse the pumpkin seeds and shredded coconut into small crumbs.
6. Transfer the crumbs to a medium-sized bowl and add the remaining crust ingredients.
7. Combine all ingredients into a thick dough and divide this mixture into six equal-sized balls.
8. Put one ball into each of the cupcake liners, pressing and flattening the balls into a crust at the bottom of each cupcake liner.
9. Transfer the tin into the freezer and prepare the filling.
10. Heat a medium-sized saucepan over medium heat and add the coconut oil. Remove the saucepan from the heat once the coconut oil has melted.
11. Put the melted coconut oil, almond butter, coconut cream, lemon juice, organic soy protein, and a pinch of salt to the (uncleaned) food processor or blender. Process these ingredients until well combined with a smooth and creamy texture.
12. Add the optional xanthan gum and stevia. Xanthan gum will help thicken the cheesecake fat bombs, while the stevia will add a sweeter flavor. Use slightly more or less stevia to taste.
13. Take the cupcake tin out of the freezer and top all crusts with filling. Make sure to divide the filling equally among the 6 cups with a tablespoon.
14. Transfer the tin back into the fridge until the cups are firm.
15. Serve the cheesecake cups at room temperature and enjoy!
16. Alternatively, store the cups in the fridge inside an airtight container and consume within 5 days.

# 17. Cashew Cocoa Bombs

Serves: 10 | Prepping Time: ~30 min |

**Nutrition Information**
(per serving)
- Calories: 455.5 kcal
- Net Carbs: 6.7 g.
- Fat: 42.5 g.
- Protein: 10.6 g.
- Fiber: 5.3 g.
- Sugar: 1.8 g.

## INGREDIENTS:
- 1 cup coconut oil
- 1 cup almond butter
- ¼ cup coconut flour
- ¼ cup cocoa powder
- ¼ cup organic soy protein
  (chocolate flavor)
- Pinch of salt
- 1 cup raw cashews (unsalted)

Total number of ingredients: 7

## METHOD:

1. Heat a medium-sized saucepan over medium heat and add the coconut oil and almond butter.
2. Stir occasionally until the oil has melted and the ingredients are combined.
3. Pour the mixture into a medium-sized bowl and, while the mixture is still warm, stir in the remaining ingredients except the cashews. Make sure all ingredients are well combined.
4. Transfer the bowl into the freezer until the dough has become firm. This should take around 15 minutes.
5. Crush the cashews into small pieces by using a coffee grinder, food processor, or blender. Spread the crushed cashew bits over a large plate.
6. Make sure that the dough is firm before making the fat bombs.
7. Take 1 tablespoon of the firm dough mixture and roll it into a ball. Roll the ball in the crushed cashews and transfer it onto a baking tray or plate. Repeat this step for all 10 balls.
8. Put the baking tray in the fridge for a few minutes to allow the bombs to firm up.
9. Take the tray out of the fridge, serve the cashew cocoa bombs and enjoy!
10. Alternatively, store the bombs in the fridge using an airtight container and consume within 6 days.

# 18. Cinnamon-Vanilla Bites

**Nutrition Information**
(per serving)
- Calories: 249.5 kcal
- Net Carbs: 1.1 g.
- Fat: 26.2 g.
- Protein: 2.1 g.
- Fiber: 1 g.
- Sugar: 0.6 g.

## INGREDIENTS:
- 1 cup coconut oil
- 1 cup cocoa butter
- 6 tbsp. almond butter
- 2 tsp. cinnamon
- 1 tsp. vanilla extract
- ¼ cup organic soy protein
  (vanilla flavor)
- 2 tbsp. water
- ½ cup dark chocolate
  (85% cocoa or higher, crushed)

Total number of ingredients: 8

## METHOD:

1. Line a large baking tray with parchment paper and set it aside.
2. In a medium-sized bowl, mix all the ingredients together. Make sure everything is incorporated and no lumps remain in the dough. Add some additional water if the dough is too thick.
3. Make sure the dough is spreadable and transfer it onto the baking tray. Spread the mixture into a large rectangular chunk.
4. Transfer the baking tray to the freezer and allow to set for about 15 minutes.
5. Fill a small saucepan with water and put it over medium heat. Place a smaller, heat-resistant metal container inside the water and put the crushed chocolate into it.
6. Melt the chocolate au bain-marie (in the bowl in the water). Be careful to keep any water from getting in the chocolate. Make sure the chocolate doesn't boil because it will ruin the flavor.
7. Take the baking tray out of the freezer and cut the dough into 10 or 20 squares.
8. Using a fork, dip each square into the molten chocolate. Repeat this for all the cinnamon-vanilla bites, putting each one back onto the baking tray.
9. Refrigerate the squares for about 15 minutes, until the chocolate coating has firmed up. Serve and enjoy!
10. Alternatively, store the bites in the fridge using an airtight container and consume within 6 days.

# 19. Green Tea & Ginger Cups ⊚

Serves: 6 | Prepping Time: ~40 min |

**Nutrition Information**
(per serving)
- Calories: 376 kcal
- Net Carbs: 1.65 g.
- Fat: 40.4 g.
- Protein: 1.3 g.
- Fiber: 0.6 g.
- Sugar: 0.3 g.

## INGREDIENTS:
- 1 cup coconut oil
- 2 tbsp. almond butter
- 2-inch piece of ginger (finely grated)
- 1 tbsp. low-carb maple syrup
- 4 tbsp. matcha green tea powder
- Pinch of Himalayan salt
- Optional: ½ tsp. stevia powder

Total number of ingredients: 7

## METHOD:

1. Line a cupcake tin with six cupcake papers and set it aside.
2. Heat a medium-sized saucepan over low heat and add the coconut oil.
3. Once the coconut oil has become soft and spreadable, remove the saucepan from the heat and transfer the oil to a medium-sized bowl.
4. Add the remaining ingredients and stir until all ingredients are combined and no lumps remain. Blend in the optional stevia powder if you prefer a sweeter flavor. Use slightly more or less stevia to taste.
5. Divide the mixture among the six cupcake papers and transfer the tin to the freezer.
6. After 30 minutes, take the cupcake tin out, serve and enjoy!
7. Alternatively, store the green tea cups in the fridge using an airtight container and consume within 5 days.

# 20. Sweet & Nutty Fudge ⓧ ⓧ

Serves: 12 | Prepping Time: ~35 min |

**Nutrition Information**
(per serving)
- Calories: 240 kcal
- Net Carbs: 3.5 g.
- Fat: 23.7 g.
- Protein: 2.5 g.
- Fiber: 3 g.
- Sugar: 2.45 g.

## INGREDIENTS:
- ½ cup coconut oil
- ½ cup coconut butter
- 1/3 cup unsweetened almond milk
- 1 cup shredded coconut (unsweetened)
- ¼ cup brazil nuts
- ¼ cup pumpkin seeds (raw)
- ½ cup raw cashews (unsalted)
- 2 tbsp. organic soy protein
  (chocolate flavor)
- 3 dates (pitted)
- Pinch of Himalayan salt

Total number of ingredients: 10

## METHOD:

1. Line a baking tray with parchment paper and set it aside.
2. Heat a medium-sized saucepan over low heat and add the coconut oil and coconut butter.
3. Once the coconut oil and coconut butter have become soft, remove the saucepan from the heat and transfer its contents to a blender or food processor.
4. Add the remaining ingredients and pulse the mixture into a thick, spreadable batter. Small chunks of ingredients are fine.
5. Transfer the batter onto the baking tray and spread it out into a large square.
6. Put the baking tray in the freezer for at least 20 minutes.
7. When the fudge has become firm, cut it into 12 squares, serve and enjoy!
8. Alternatively, store the fudge in the fridge using an airtight container and consume within 6 days.

# 21. Espresso Protein Cups

Serves: 9 | Prepping Time: ~40 min |

**Nutrition Information**
(per serving)
- Calories: 245 kcal
- Net Carbs: 2.7 g.
- Fat: 22.2 g.
- Protein: 7.9 g.
- Fiber: 2.7 g.
- Sugar: 0.9 g.

## INGREDIENTS:
- 1 cup almond butter
  (or cashew butter)
- ¼ cup coconut oil
- ¼ cup organic soy protein
  (chocolate flavor)
- 2 tsp. instant espresso powder
  (or instant coffee powder)
- ½ tsp. stevia powder
- Optional: 1 tbsp. full-fat coconut milk

Total number of ingredients: 6

## METHOD:

1. Line a cupcake tin with nine cupcake liners and set it aside.
2. Heat a medium-sized saucepan over medium-low heat and add all the ingredients, including the optional coconut milk.
3. Incorporate all ingredients while stirring constantly. If desired, add more espresso powder, stevia powder, coconut milk, and/or soy protein to taste.
4. Divide the mixture equally into the nine cupcake liners and transfer the tin to the freezer.
5. After 30 minutes, take the cupcake tin out, serve the cups and enjoy!
6. Alternatively, store the espresso protein cups in the fridge using an airtight container and consume within 7 days.

*Tip: This makes a perfect ketogenic snack to start the day with, thanks to the natural caffeine from coffee!*

# 22. Blackberry Peanut Squares

Serves: 8 | Prepping Time: ~30 min |

**Nutrition Information**
(per serving)
- Calories: 251 kcal
- Net Carbs: 5.6 g.
- Fat: 21.3 g.
- Protein: 8.7 g.
- Fiber: 2.7 g.
- Sugar: 3.5 g.

## INGREDIENTS:
- 1 cup peanut butter (page 30)
- ½ cup coconut cream
- ½ cup blackberries (fresh or frozen)
- 1 tbsp. lemon juice
- ½ tsp. vanilla extract

Total number of ingredients: 5

## METHOD:

1. Line a baking tray with parchment paper and set it aside.
2. Heat a medium-sized saucepan over medium-low heat and add all the ingredients. Slowly heat the ingredients while stirring occasionally. Fresh berries can be incorporated, but should not be heated beyond 110°F/45°C.
3. Transfer the mixture to a food processor or blender and process until all ingredients are incorporated and smooth.
4. Spread the mixture into a square form on the baking tray.
5. Transfer the baking tray to the freezer and allow the chunk to set. This should take about 30 minutes.
6. Take out the baking tray, remove the chunk, and cut it into 8 equal squares.
7. Serve the blackberry peanut squares and enjoy!
8. Alternatively, store the squares in the fridge using an airtight container and consume within 4 days.

Tip: Substitute the blackberries for strawberries or loganberries!

# 23. 3-Ingredient Berry Bites

Serves: 6 | Prepping Time: ~35 min |

**Nutrition Information**
(per serving)
- Calories: 341 kcal
- Net Carbs: 1 g.
- Fat: 37.3 g.
- Protein: 0 g.
- Fiber: 0.75 g.
- Sugar: 0.8 g.

## INGREDIENTS:
- 1 cup coconut oil
- ½ cup mixed berries (fresh or frozen)
- 1 tsp. vanilla extract

Total number of ingredients: 3

## METHOD:

1. Line a baking tray with parchment paper and set it aside.
2. Heat a medium-sized saucepan over medium-low heat and add the coconut oil.
3. Once the oil has melted, take the saucepan off the heat and transfer its contents to a food processor or blender.
4. Add the berries and the vanilla extract and process until all ingredients are incorporated and smooth.
5. Spread the mixture into a square form on the baking tray.
6. Transfer the baking tray to the freezer and allow the chunk to set. This should take about 25 minutes.
7. Take out the baking tray, remove the chunk, and cut it into 6 equal pieces.
8. Serve the berry bites and enjoy!
9. Alternatively, store the bites in the fridge using an airtight container and consume within 4 days.

*Tip: Add pomegranates, cherries or strawberries to the mix!*

# 24. Matcha Coconut Balls

Serves: 16 | Prepping Time: ~25 min |

**Nutrition Information**
(per serving)
- Calories: 262 kcal
- Net Carbs: 2.2 g.
- Fat: 27.7 g.
- Protein: 0.36 g.
- Fiber: 3.1 g.
- Sugar: 1.5 g.

## INGREDIENTS:
- 1 cup coconut oil
- 1 cup coconut butter
- ½ cup full-fat coconut milk (refrigerated)
- 1 ½ tsp. matcha green tea powder
- 1 tsp. vanilla extract
- 2 tbsp. organic lemon zest
- Pinch of sea salt
- 1 cup shredded coconut

Total number of ingredients: 8

## METHOD:

1. Add all the ingredients except the shredded coconut to a medium-sized bowl. Microwave the bowl for a few seconds until the coconut oil has melted.
2. Use a mixer to combine all ingredients in the bowl.
3. Cover the bowl and transfer it to the refrigerator.
4. Line a baking tray with parchment paper and spread the shredded coconut over it.
5. After one hour, take the bowl out of the fridge and use a tablespoon to form 16 balls.
6. Coat each ball in the shredded coconut and line them up on a baking tray.
7. Transfer the tray into the fridge for another 15 minutes.
8. Serve the matcha coconut balls and enjoy!
9. Alternatively, store the balls in the fridge using an airtight container and consume within 12 days.

*Tip: Can't get enough of the matcha? Coat the balls in both the shredded coconut and some additional matcha green tea powder!*

# Conclusion

I would like to thank you for purchasing this book and taking the time to read it. I hope that it has been helpful to you!

The Ketogenic Vegan diet is very beneficial for your health and stamina. The combination of these two diets is one of the best you can find for your physical well-being and mental performance. Commit to it and you will reap the benefits!

Did you like this book? Then don't forget to leave a review on Amazon!

This way other readers can get inspired too.

**Love,**

Lydia

**Congratulations with your responsible and health-conscious decision to read my book.**

*I'm very excited for you!*

I offer my readers an *exclusive* opportunity to become part of my keto circle. Dozens of people are already inside and enjoying *extra* (vegan & vegetarian) ketogenic recipes and support on their journey to fat-fueled cooking, more energy and weight loss.

Join a growing number of 'plant-ketoers' and become part of my circle!

**https://forms.aweber.com/form/96/2128265096.htm**

You'll get *'The Keto Vegetarian: 8 Reader-Exclusive Low-Carb, Plant-Based, Egg & Dairy Recipes'* as a welcome gift!

Subscribe to my newsletter and join dozens of people with similar aims and ethics.

**https://forms.aweber.com/form/96/2128265096.htm**

*(I absolutely hate spam and will never email you more than twice a week.)*

As a member of my keto circle, you will receive some of my latest recipes, exclusive opportunities to get new releases free of charge, and more...!

As a member of my keto circle, you can also always reach out for personal questions!

Check out my Facebook page:

**www.facebook.com/veganvegetarianketo**

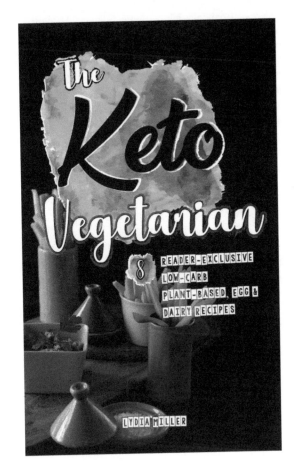

And our Facebook group:

**www.facebook.com/groups/veganvegetarianketo**

Where you get inspired, share results with other 'plant-ketoers' and stay motivated on your keto journey!

See you inside!

*Lydia*

# Sources

1. https://www.ncbi.nlm.nih.gov/pmc/articles/PMC5466942/
   https://www.ncbi.nlm.nih.gov/pmc/articles/PMC4991921/
2. https://www.ncbi.nlm.nih.gov/pmc/articles/PMC5466942/
   https://www.ncbi.nlm.nih.gov/pmc/articles/PMC3662288/
3. https://www.ncbi.nlm.nih.gov/pmc/articles/PMC5409832/
4. https://www.ncbi.nlm.nih.gov/pmc/articles/PMC5452247/
5. http://www.jlr.org/content/30/11/1727.abstract
6. https://www.nature.com/articles/0802369
7. https://www.ncbi.nlm.nih.gov/pmc/articles/PMC3945587/
8. https://www.ncbi.nlm.nih.gov/pubmed/9416027
9. https://www.livestrong.com/article/267249-amino-acid-supplements-for-women/
   https://www.ncbi.nlm.nih.gov/pmc/articles/PMC4935284/
10. https://www.ncbi.nlm.nih.gov/pmc/articles/PMC4935284/
11. https://www.nutrition.org.uk/nutritionscience/nutrients-food-and-ingredients/protein.html?limit=1&start=2
12. Dietetics Manual by Jean Lederer
13. https://www.aafp.org/afp/2009/0101/p43.html
14. https://academic.oup.com/ajcn/article/101/6/1317S/4564491
15. https://www.ncbi.nlm.nih.gov/pmc/articles/PMC3449675/
16. http://www.who.int/nutrition/publications/nutrientrequirements/WHO_TRS_935/en
17. http://www.dummies.com/health/nutrition/what-are-simple-carbohydrates-complex-carbohydrates-and-dietary-fiber
18. http://www.diabetes.org/food-and-fitness/food/what-can-i-eat/understanding-carbohydrates/glycemic-index-and-diabetes.html
19. https://www.cambridge.org/core/services/aop-cambridge-core/content/view/AF44097B0E9C4FF9BD44F1D55CD353D6/
    S0007114514002931a.pdf/does_cooking_with_vegetable_oils_increase_the_risk_of_chronic_diseases_a_systematic_review.pdf
    https://www.sciencedirect.com/science/article/pii/S0278691510004941?via%3Dihub
20. https://www.ncbi.nlm.nih.gov/pubmed/29511019
21. https://www.ncbi.nlm.nih.gov/pmc/articles/PMC4365303/
22. https://www.ncbi.nlm.nih.gov/pmc/articles/PMC4892314/
23. https://www.ncbi.nlm.nih.gov/pmc/articles/PMC5646809/
    https://www.ncbi.nlm.nih.gov/pmc/articles/PMC2974200/
24. https://www.ncbi.nlm.nih.gov/pubmed/12442909
25. https://www.ncbi.nlm.nih.gov/pmc/articles/PMC5611753/
    https://www.gbhealthwatch.com/Science-Omega3-Omega6.php
26. https://www.joslin.org/info/how_does_fiber_affect_blood_glucose_levels.html
27. fiberfacts.org/fibers-count-calories-carbohydrates
28. 'A ketogenic diet as a potential novel therapeutic intervention in amyotrophic lateral sclerosis' by Zhao et al
    'Ketogenic diet protects dopaminergic neurons against 6-OHDA neurotoxicity via up-regulating glutathione in a rat model of Parkinson's disease' by Cheng et al
    'The ketogenic diet: metabolic influences on brain excitability and epilepsy' by Lutas & Yellen

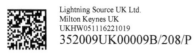